Sinsemilla

MARIJUANA FLOWERS

BY

JIM RICHARDSON

PHOTOGRAPHY

BY

ARIK WOODS

AND/OR PRESS
BERKELEY, CALIFORNIA
1976

The publisher does not advocate breaking the law.
This material is presented in the spirit of information
to be made available to the public.

Copyright © 1976 by Jim Richardson, Arik Woods and Jay Bogart

ISBN 0-915904-23-3   FIRST PRINTING

published and distributed by
AND/OR PRESS
BOX 2246
BERKELEY, CALIFORNIA 94702

This book is dedicated to the Hermit.

PREFACE

Sinsemilla is the sweet unpollinated flowers of the female hemp plant. It is a Spanish word meaning "without seed." This book is about the genesis of the seedless marijuana plant, from the germination of the seed to the ripening of the flowers. This is a photographic study of the changing rhythms of the living plant, a tour of a sinsemilla garden through a magnifying glass. We have tried to express the delicacy and subtlety of this power plant which has come down to us from antiquity. There are many voices of the hemp and we have chosen one to tell our story.

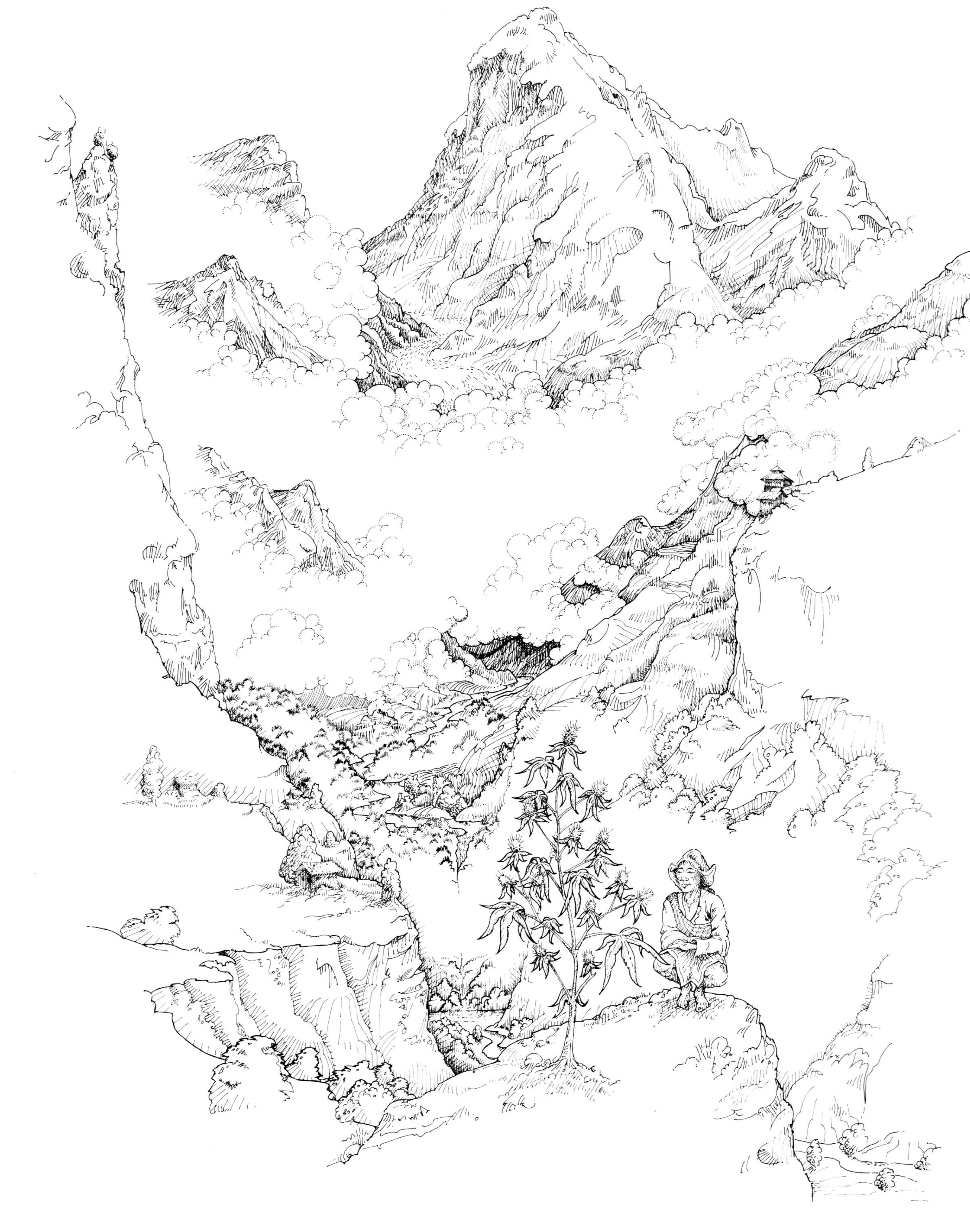

FOREWORD

SINSEMILLA

Smugglers brought me my first word of it; "and if you think this is good, you should see the incredible seedless weed that the farmers grow for themselves."

These seedless ladies are so strong, and they carry such enormous weight in buds that just a few plants can give a person, with the patience to raise them, all the joyous smoke they want from season to season.

The surprise of it is that these ladies give as much pleasure to me with the fragrance of their flowers, their color and symmetry as they give by being unquestionably the best smoke in the world.

DAVID CROSBY
July 1976

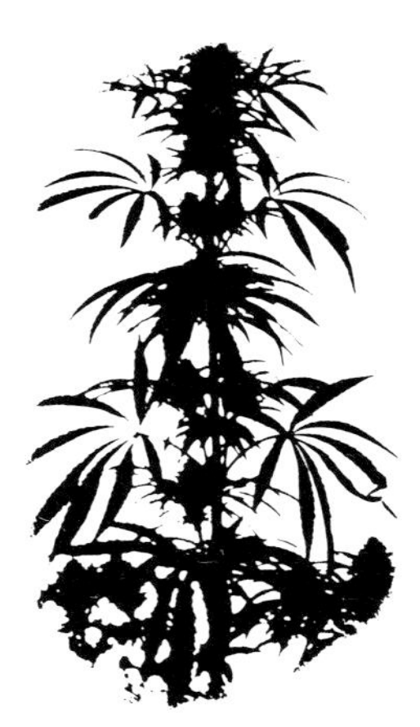

PART ONE

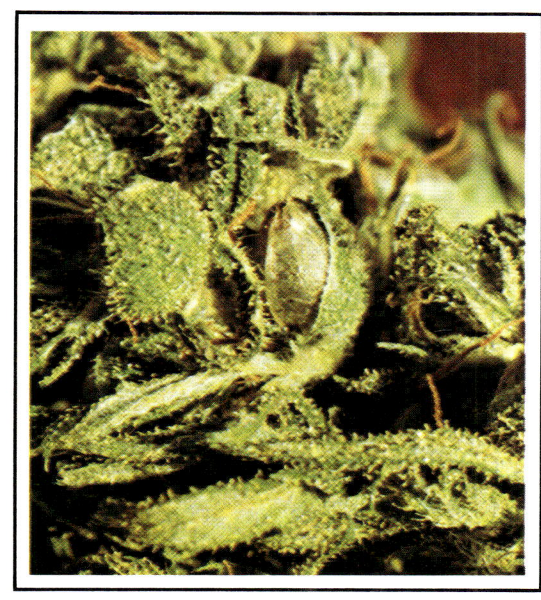

THE SEED

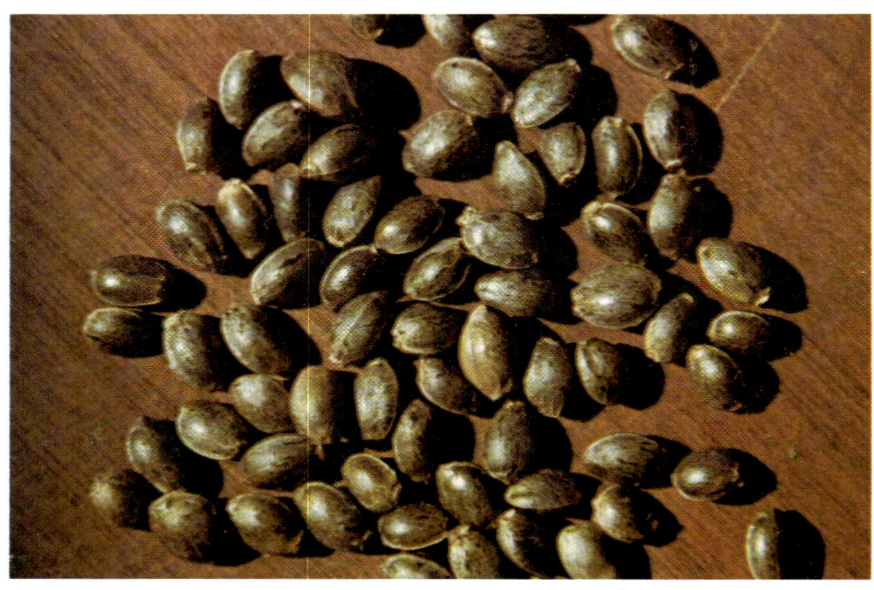

FROM THE MOTHER PLANT is born the seed: the plan of life and the hope of regenesis. From the parent plants, the seed inherits the genetic code which defines the basic physical characteristics and the essential nature of the smoke. The seed determines the potential of the plant and favorable conditions must be created which will realize this potential.

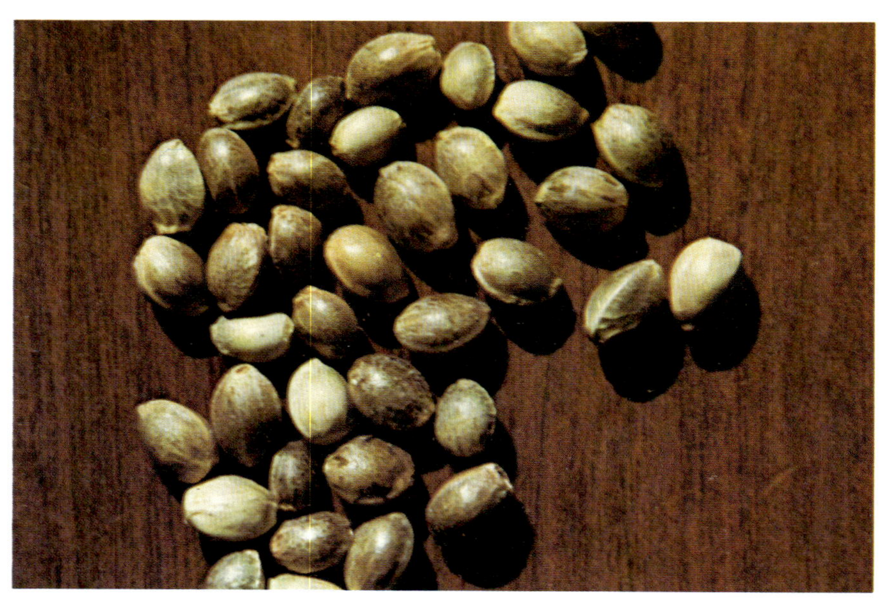

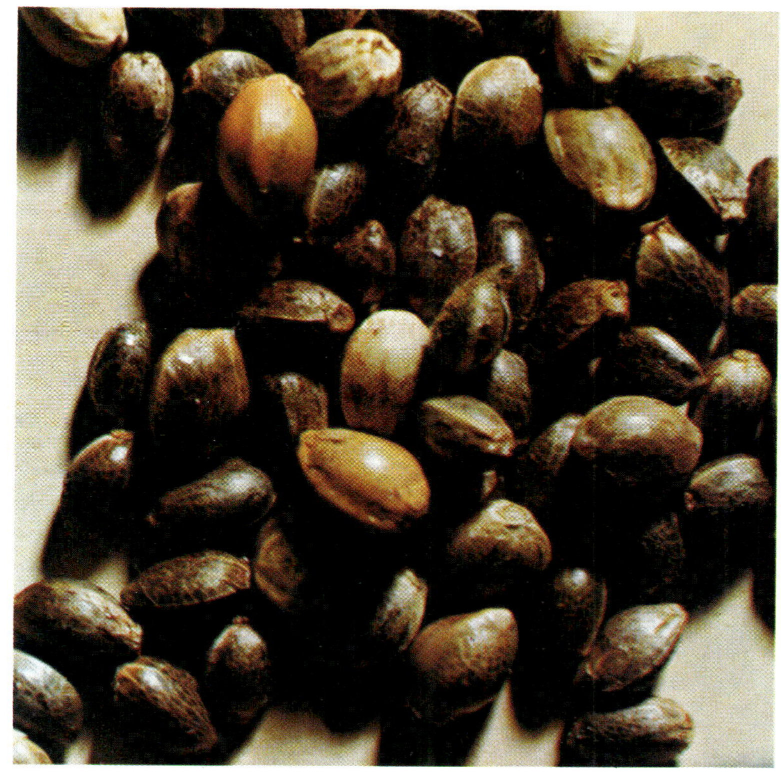

IN THE MEAT of the seed is stored the food the sprout will need to begin its life. The seed is protected by a thin wax-like coating which retards the movement of moisture into and out of the nut. When cast upon the earth in its natural cycle, the seed remains strong only a single season. But if carefully protected from moisture and heat, the seed will remain viable for a number of years.

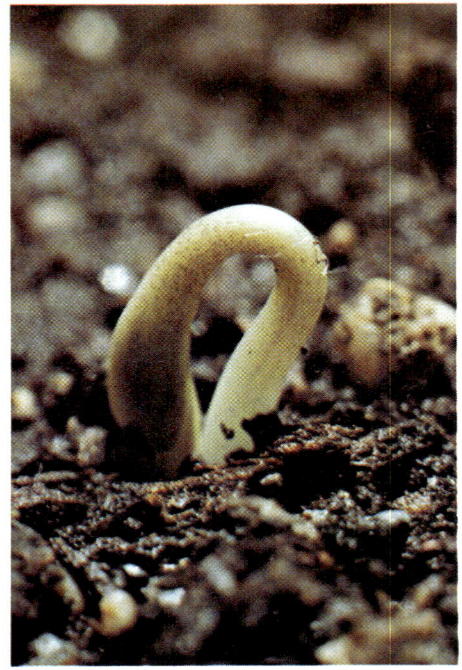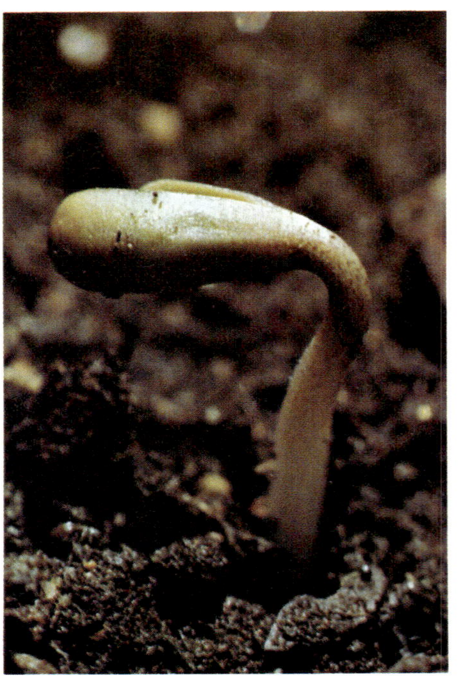

GERMINATION REQUIRES a womb-like state of warmth and moisture, preferably in darkness. The cells of the nut absorb water from the soil and soon soften and swell with life. Within a day or two the white root sprouts from the pointed end. It elongates and curves back upon itself. If the pointed end of the seed is facing upward, the root levers the seed body toward the surface in a single motion. The folded stalk breaks ground first, and pulls the soft nut from the earth as it grows upward.

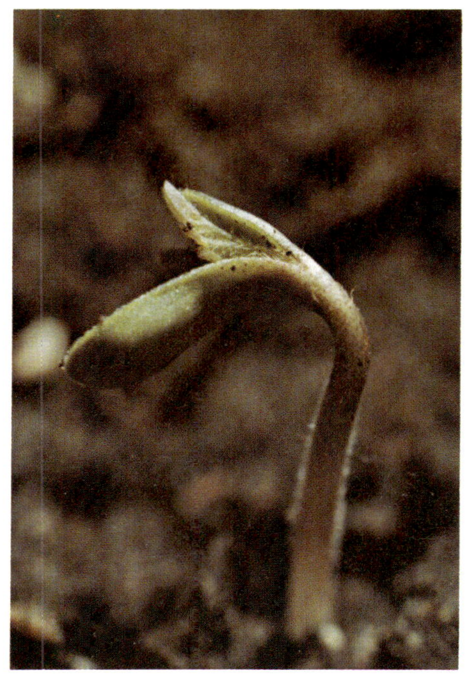 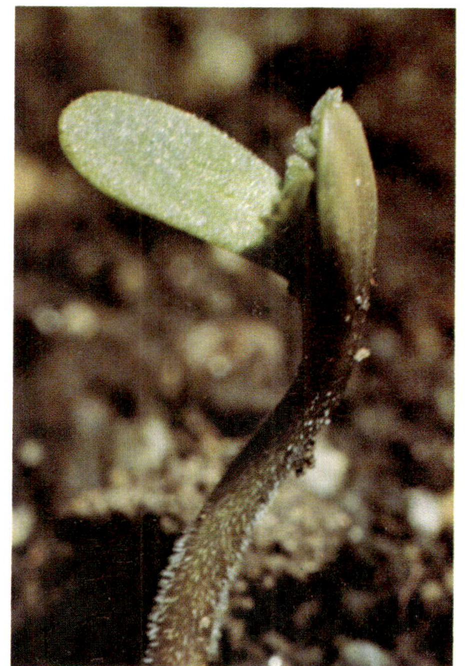

AS THE SWOLLEN NUT clears the surface, the seed covering falls away and the seed bursts in half, forming the first green leaves of the new plant. The seedling rights itself and stands erect; the root grows down and drinks from the soil. The new organism now has the ability to receive energy from the sun and create living matter.

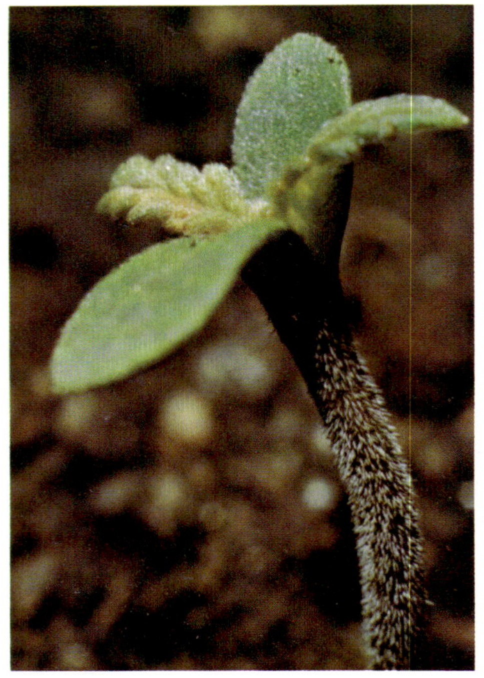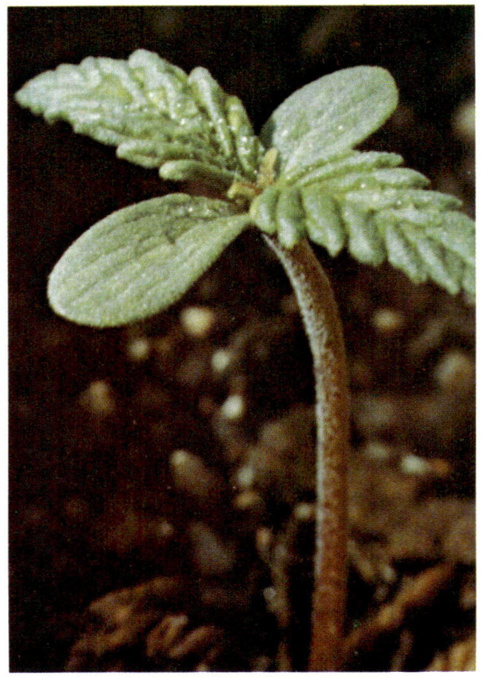

THE FIRST SERRATED LEAVES are nestled between the oval leaves. They grow rapidly, and as the stalk grows upward the next pair can soon be seen growing out of the center of the leaf cluster. In weeks to come, this basic progression will repeat itself over and over again and the plant will multiply its size thousands of times. As the plant grows upward the number of fingers in the fan increases, usually in odd increments up to eleven. In robust plants, this progression will be more rapid and the second pair may already have five parts in the fan.

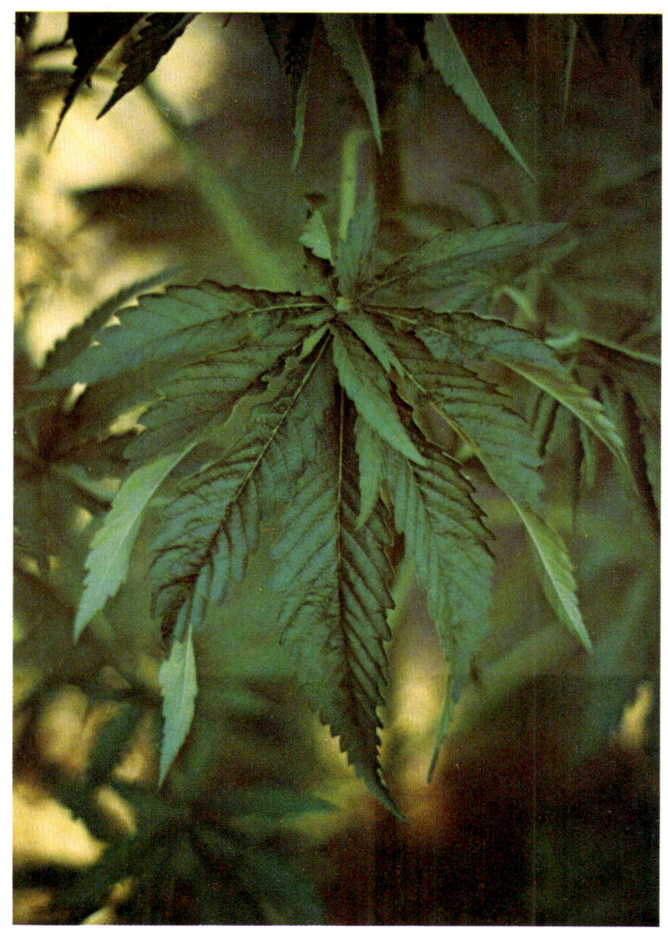

ALL DEGREES OF VARIATION occur in the leaf patterns, especially in dynamic plants. At times, the plant seems to lose all regard for order. We have found large leaves on the main stalk with up to twenty parts. These are usually in a basic fan of eleven or thirteen with the other fingers somewhat less developed and shooting randomly out of the fan. This often occurs as the plant reaches full size and seems to have no effect on the potency of the flowers.

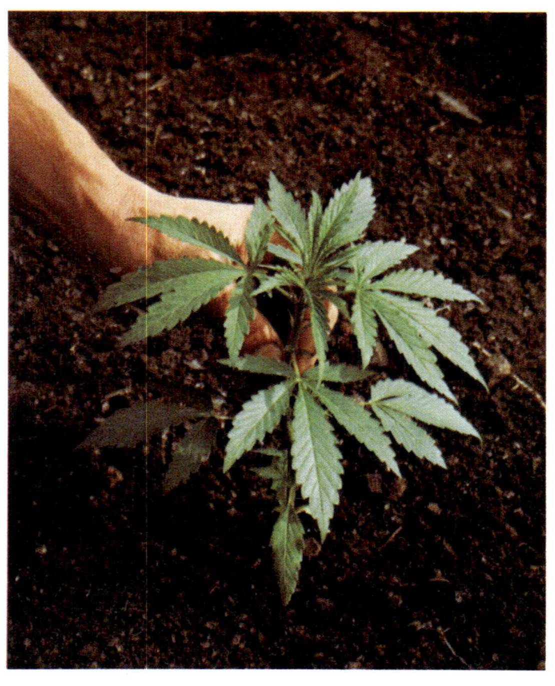

THE YOUNG SEEDLING is a perfect miniature of the full grown plant. The same patterns will repeat themselves millions of times in the life of the plant. Everything is in perfect scale. This is the same frame that in months will support pounds of resinous flower clusters.

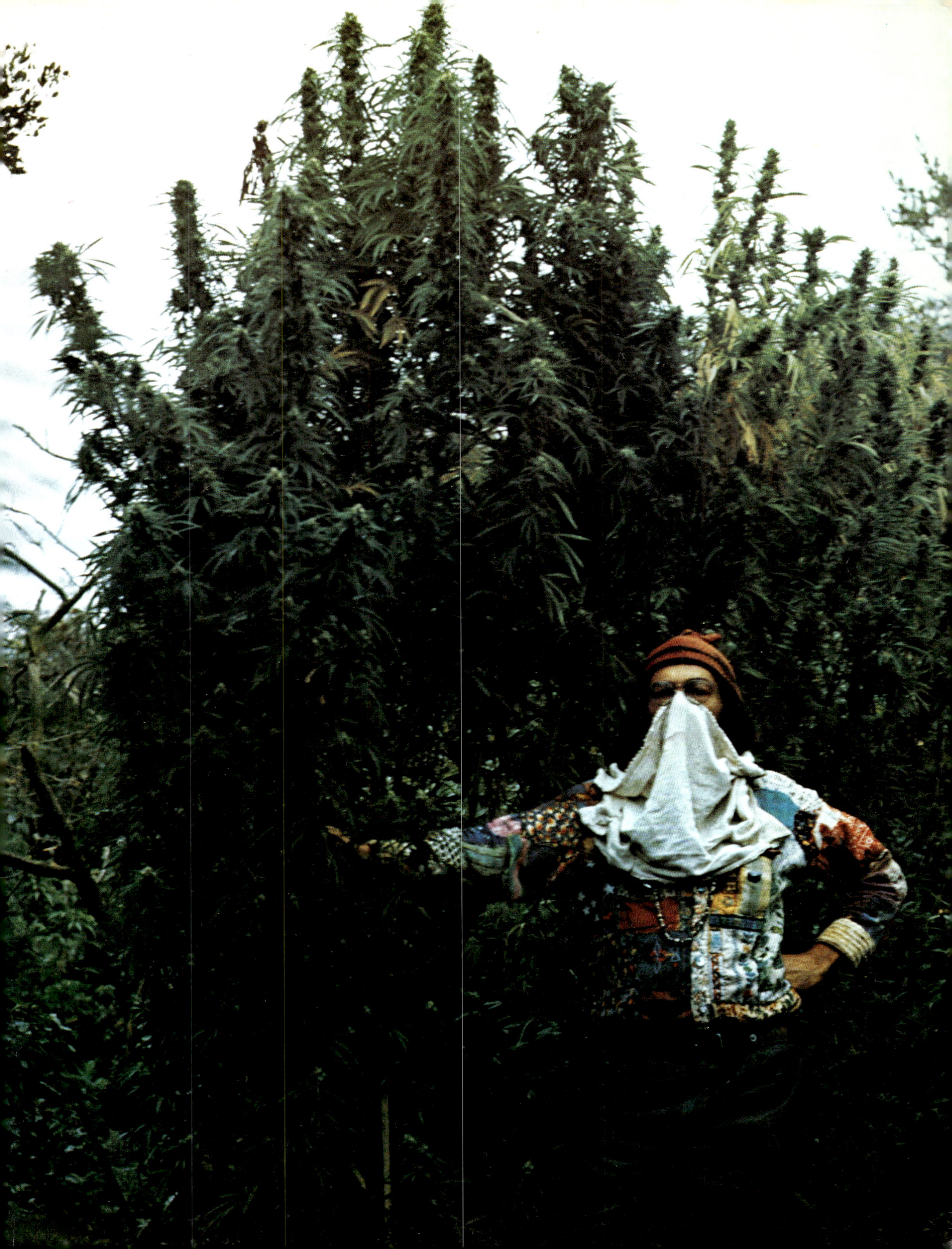

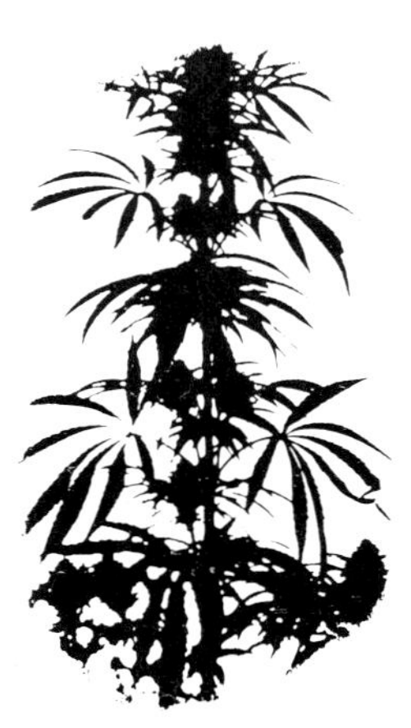

PART TWO

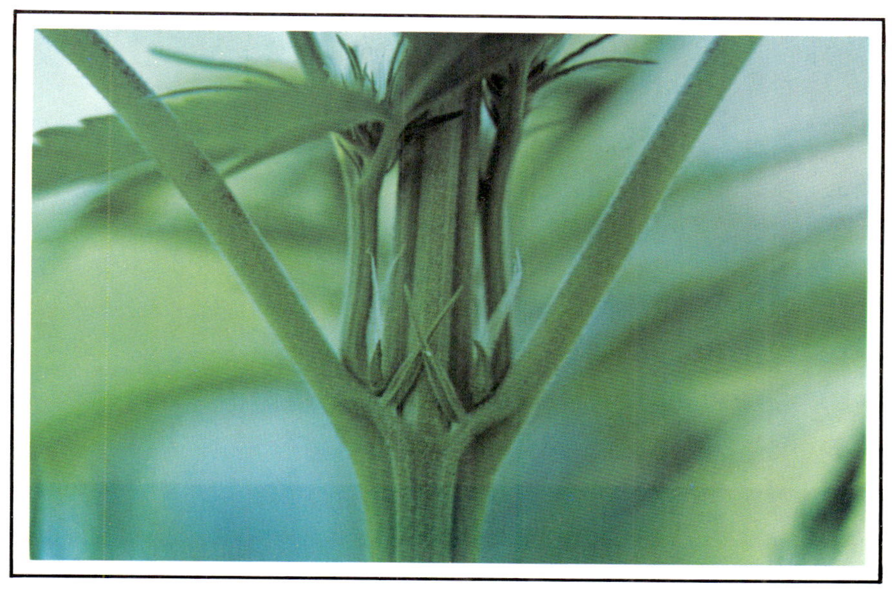

ADOLESCENCE

THE HEMP PLANT has a beautiful and intricate mechanism of reproduction. The plant is classified as dioecious: having the male and female organs on separate plants. The male flower produces the pollen, the fertilizing element. The female flower receives the pollen floating in the air and creates her seed.

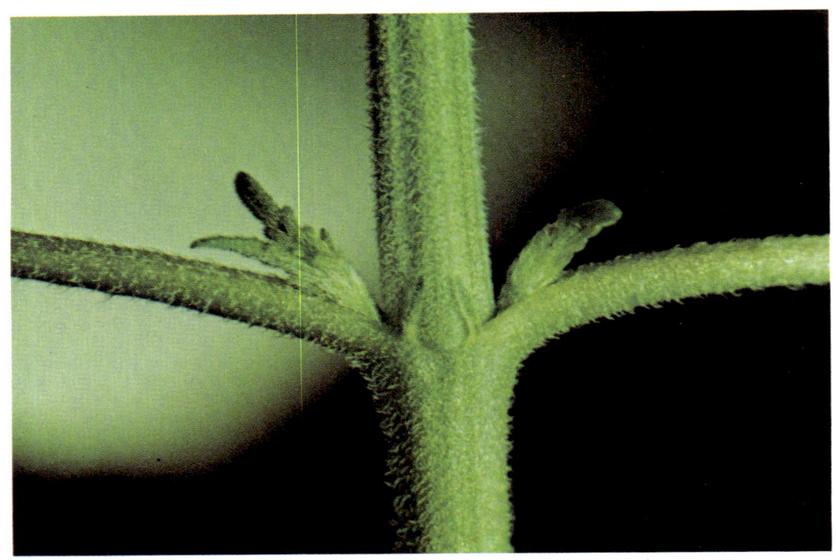

the leaf spurs at the nodes of a three-week-old seedling, long before the first flowers appear

IN SINSEMILLA, to eliminate pollination, we must identify and remove the males before their blossoms open and disperse the pollen. Sexual distinctions in the young plants cannot be determined by their shape, coloration or size. It is especially easy to confuse subtle variations in strain characteristics with sexual characteristics in adolescent plants. As we know, there is one precise method of determining gender before the true flower clusters appear on the branches of the plant.

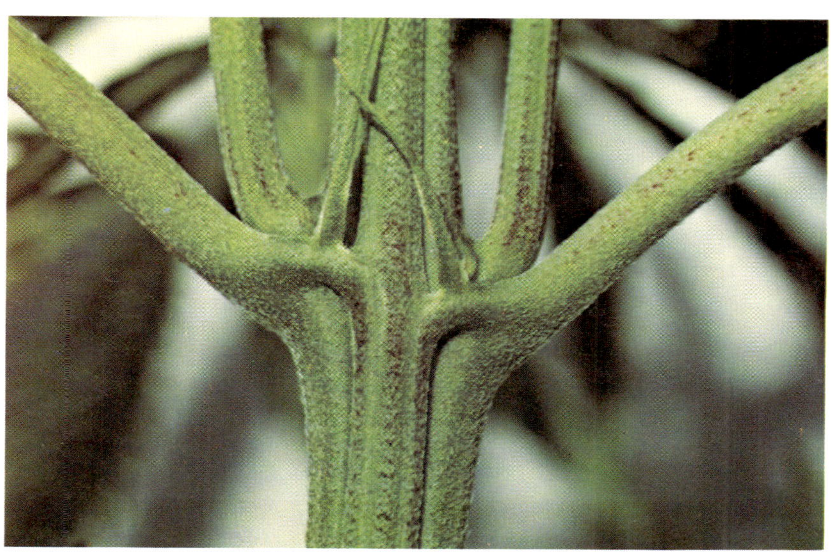

the nodes of an adolescent female
as the buds appear behind the spurs

WE MUST LOOK very closely to see where the hemp first shows gender. We look near the top of the plant, on the main stalk or on the large branches, usually at the second or third crotch below the growing tip. At the crotch, large fan leaves and branch systems shoot out from the trunk. Here on the face of the stalk occurs a swelling called a node. From the nodes grow spearlike protrusions one-fourth to one-half inch long. Where the branches grow opposite, these leaf spurs cross their tips, forming a tipi pattern against the trunk. Nestled behind the spur, in the crotch formed by the leaf stem and the main stalk, appear the first sexual organs. These single, isolated flowers can usually be seen several weeks before the true flower clusters become visible on the branches. Their cycle is identical to that of the later flowers.

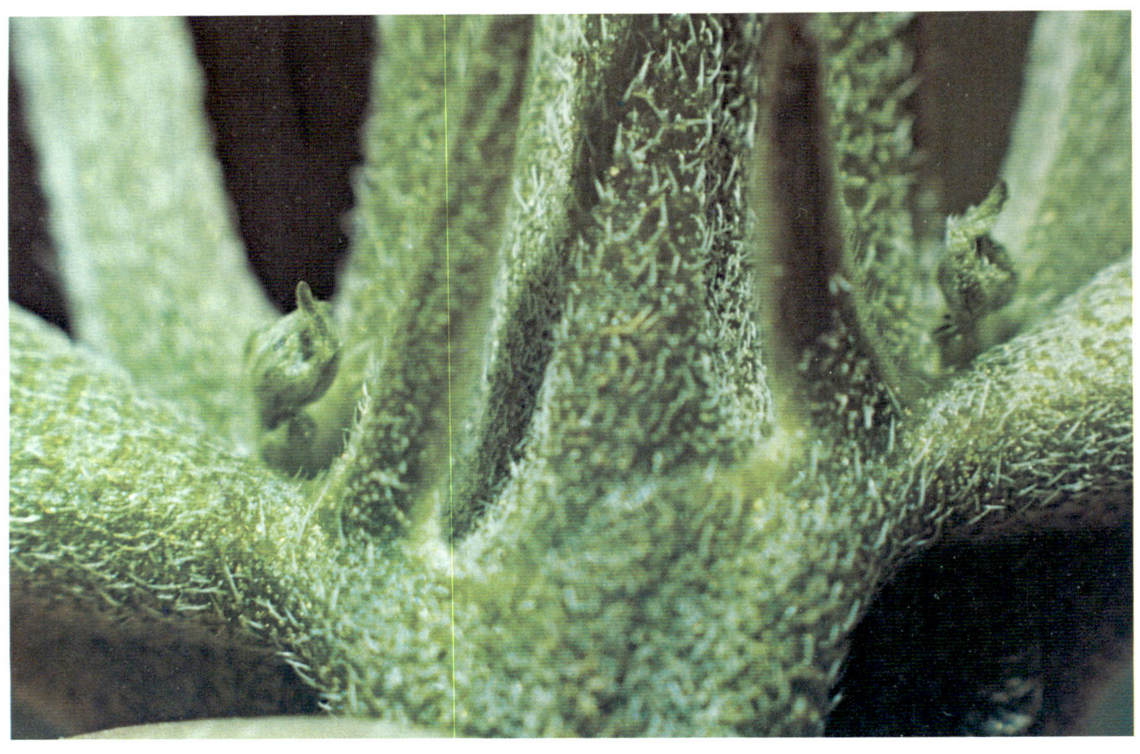

the male sac

IN THE PUBESCENT MALE we see a tiny, knob-like cluster. At first this grows straight up, but soon the knob becomes more pronounced and the organ begins to hang down, typical of the male parts.

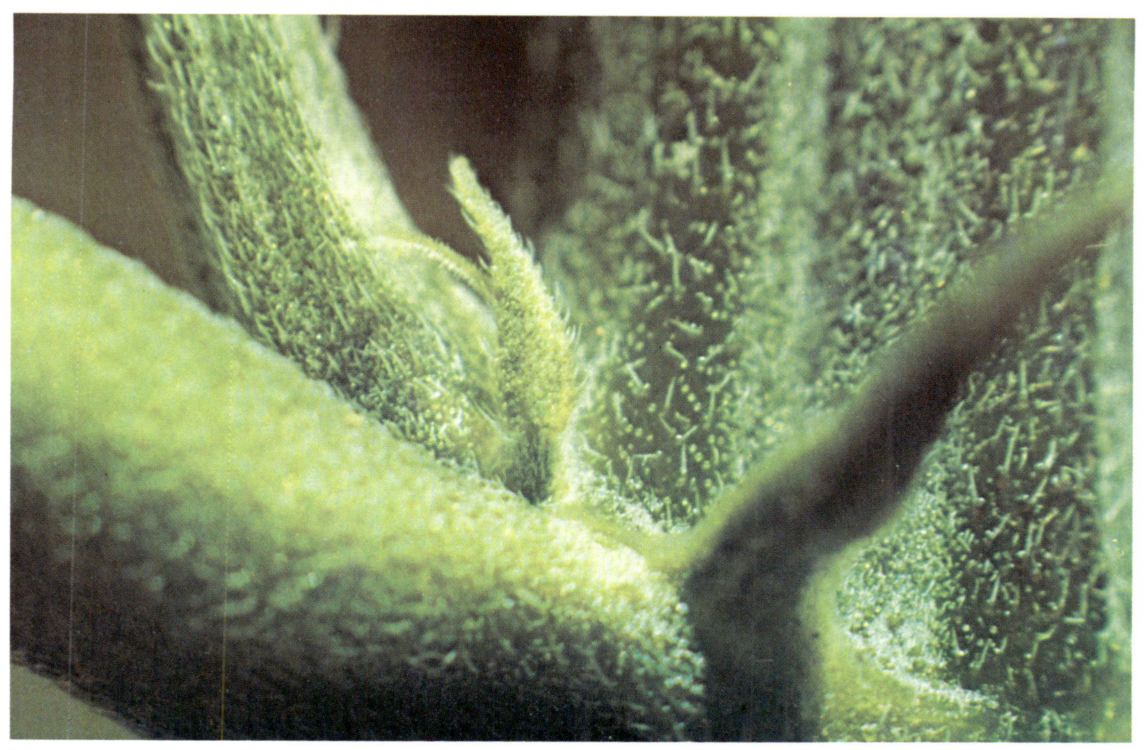

the female sheath

AT PUBERTY the female flower appears as a smooth tapering sheath, arching upward behind the leaf-spur. It begins as a pinpoint and soom grows to about half the size of the spur. At early stages, direction of growth is an important sexual distinction. The female continues to grow upward while the male tends to hang down.

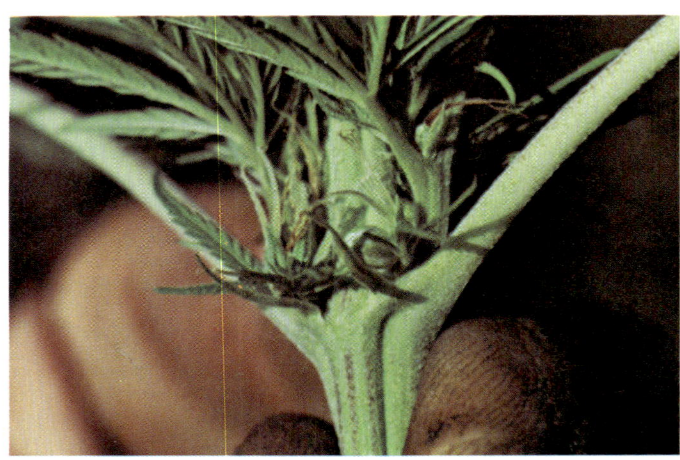

occasionally the flowers at the nodes
multiply and form clusters

THE SHEATH, which we first identify in the female, is the immature seed cover. From this soon grows the pair of white hairs characteristic of the female hemp. These are the pistils, the organs which later receive the pollen from the air. To perform this task, the pistils are covered with a thick, downy fuzz which becomes sticky with resin as the flower matures.

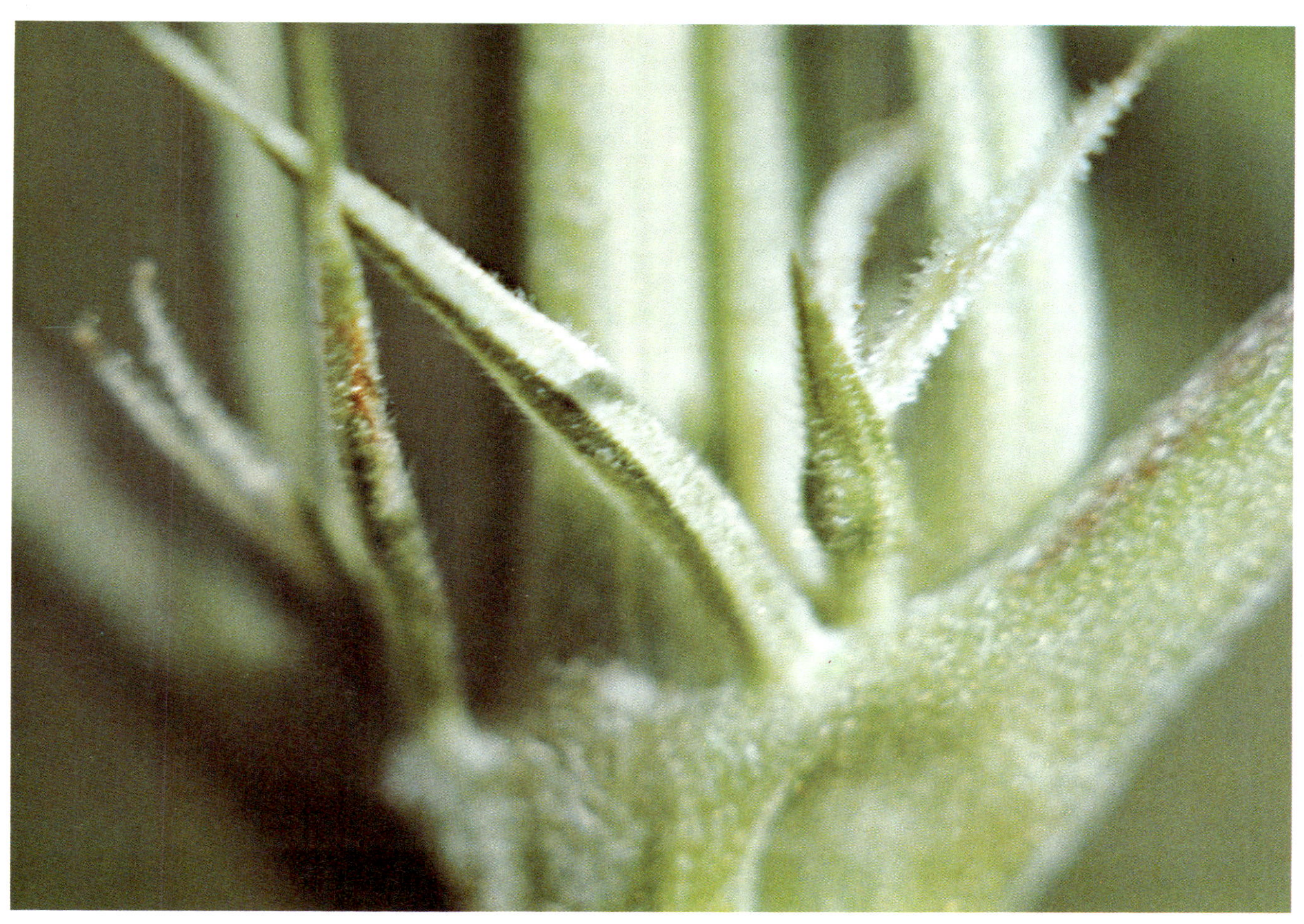

the first flower to bloom, behind the leaf-spur

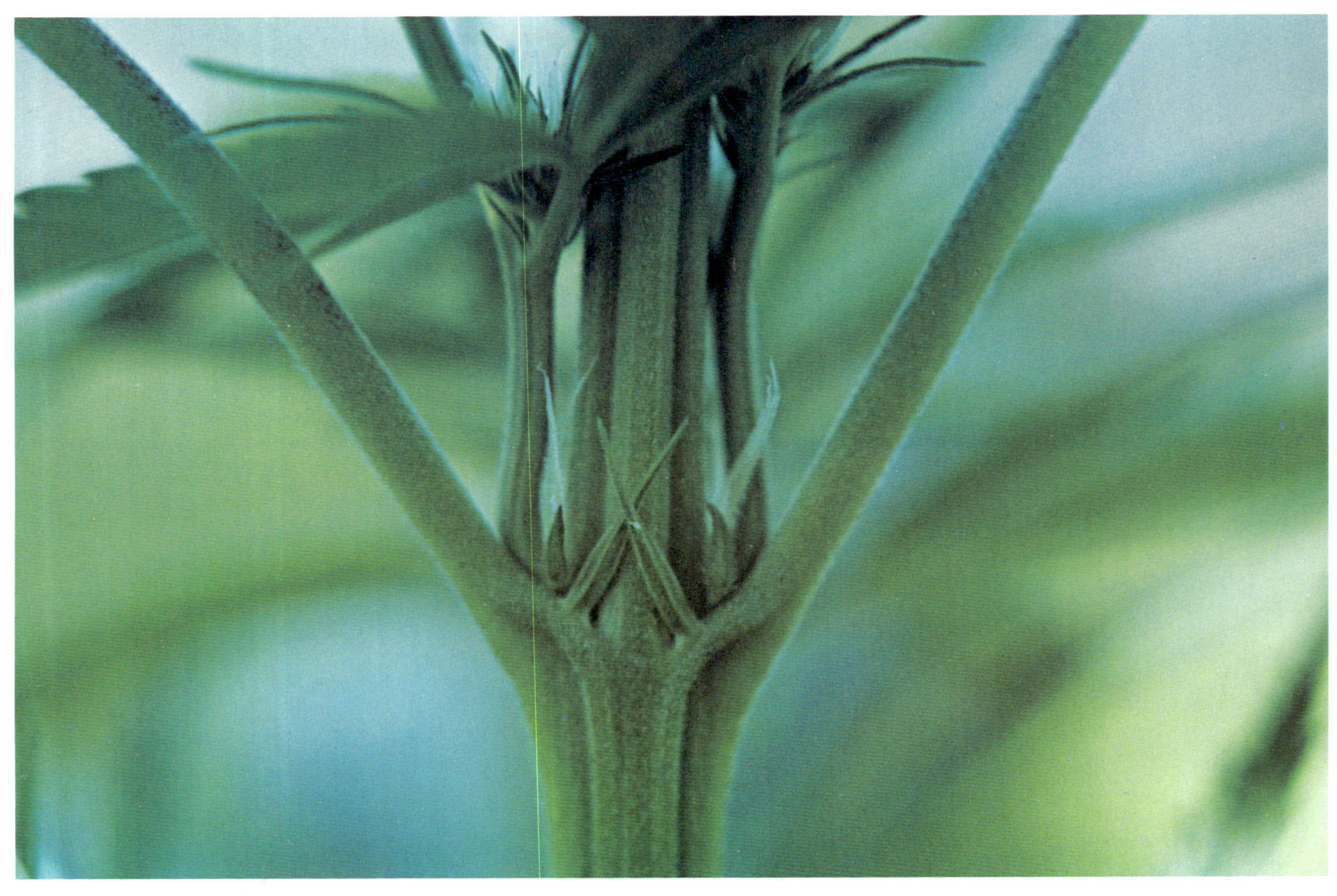

the classic female form

GIVEN A NORMAL SPRING PLANTING these preliminary organs will appear at the nodes in the height of summer, usually June to August. The size of the plants will also vary. Extremely robust plants may reach several feet by this time and may be severely overcrowding one another before the males are pulled. Variation is the rule, especially in fall and winter.

SOMETIMES THESE tiny flowers are very difficult to find, but sooner or later they do appear. Sometimes they will be apparent at every node, but sometimes the entire plant must be searched to find a lone flower. As the plant grows, more single flowers appear at the nodes and they become more obvious. At first the distinctions are incredibly subtle, but as the pistils grow out and the sacs hang down, there is no question.

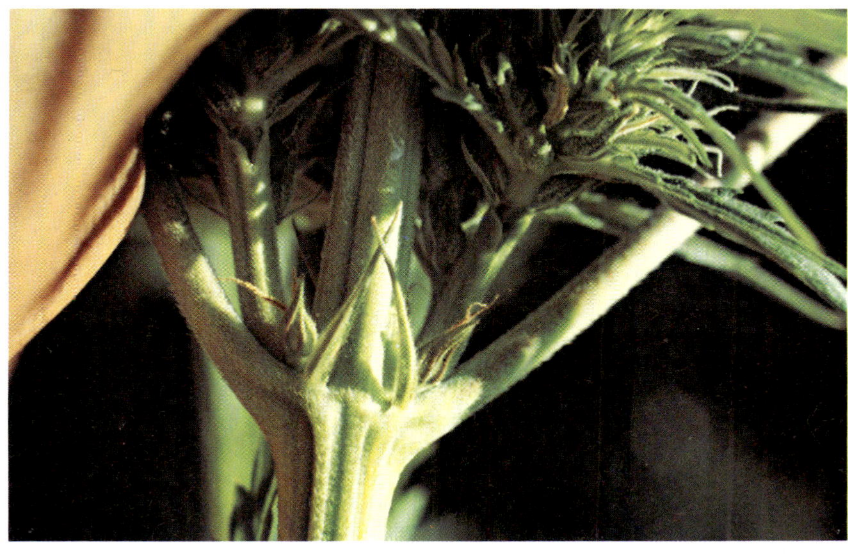

here the pistils of the preliminary flowers have passed through their cycle and the empty seed covers have developed coarse ridges

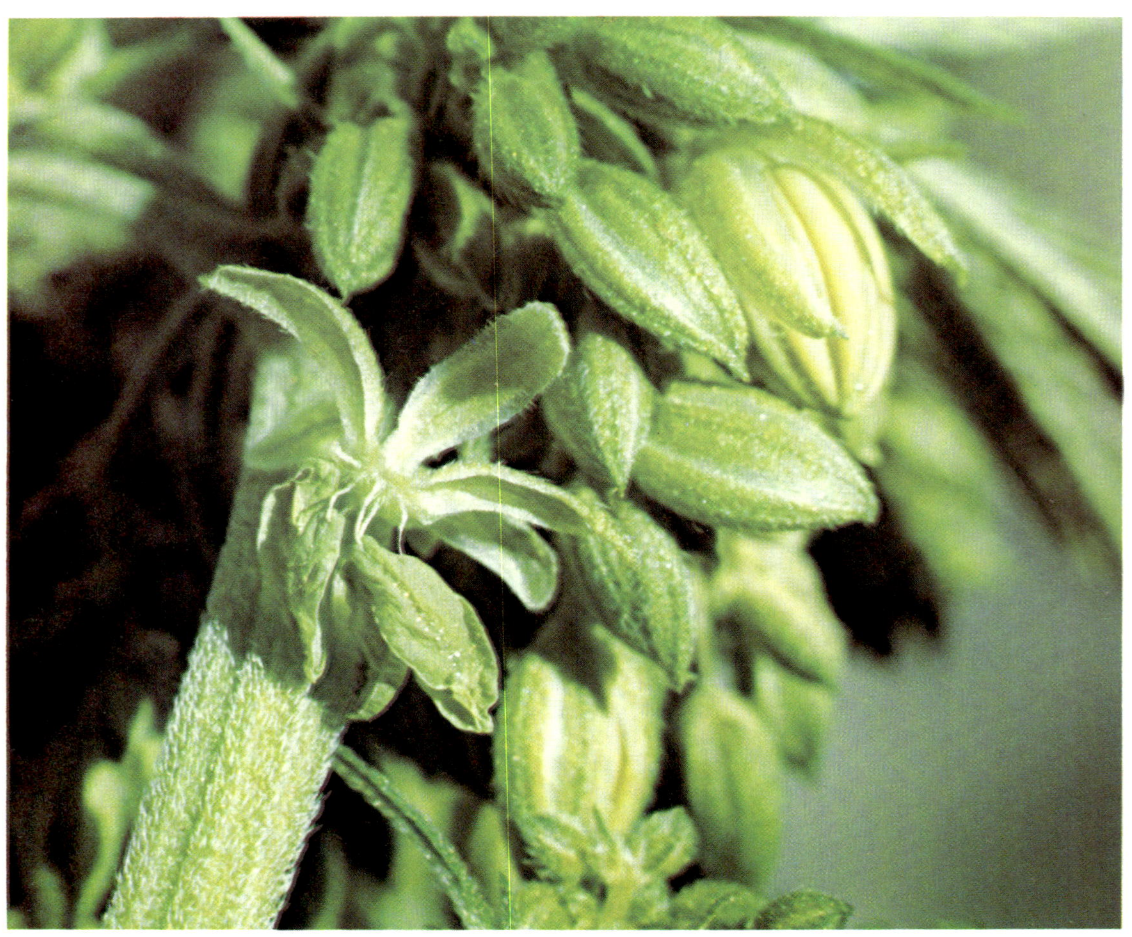

male sacs in all stages: closed, opening and spent

*(opposite) a male plant a few days
before the main pollen drop
. . . the sacs are developing rapidly*

THE MALE SAC develops longitudinal ridges and grows to more of a point. The sac swells, and at maturity the five stamens forming the sac burst apart, allowing the pollen-filled anthers to release their load into the air. The cycle of the male flower is shorter than that of the female. With the dispersal of its pollen, the male blossom is finished. The organ hangs empty.

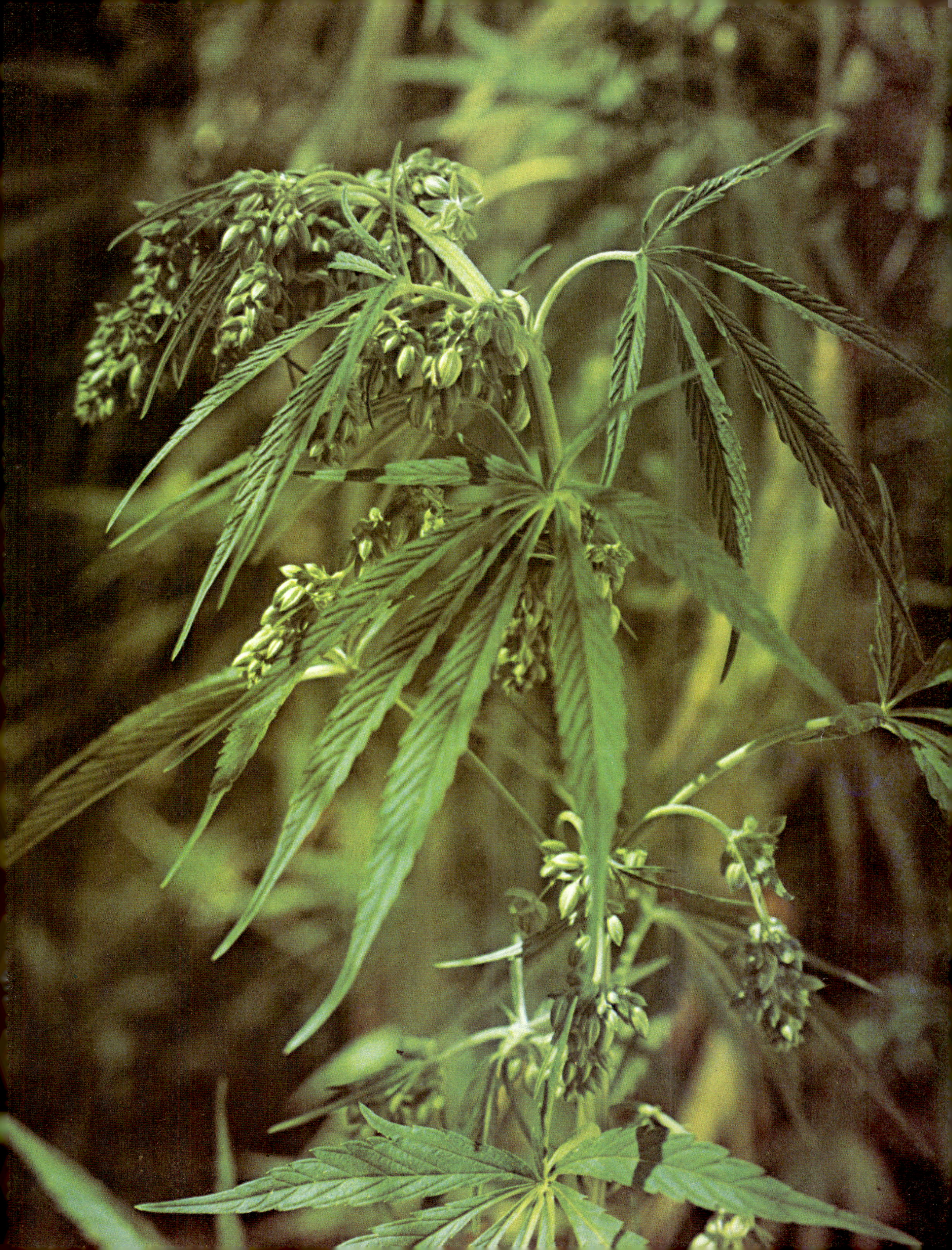

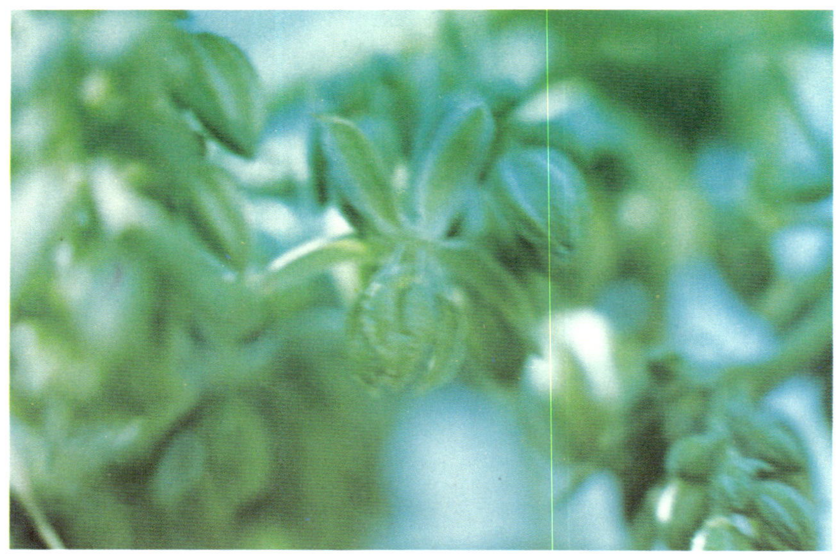

IN STRAIGHTFORWARD heterosexual plants these basic distinctions are accurate, but the cannabis does not exist in a fixed form. Under certain conditions the plant may develop as an hermaphrodite, expressing both the male and female characteristics. Organs of both sexes can be combined in single flowers and/or perfect examples of each can exist side by side in the same plant. Either sex can be dominant or the balance can be equal. Sexuality is determined by a subtle interplay of conditions. It seems that when the environment is unbalanced and threatening to the organism, more males are likely to appear and sexuality is more ambiguous.

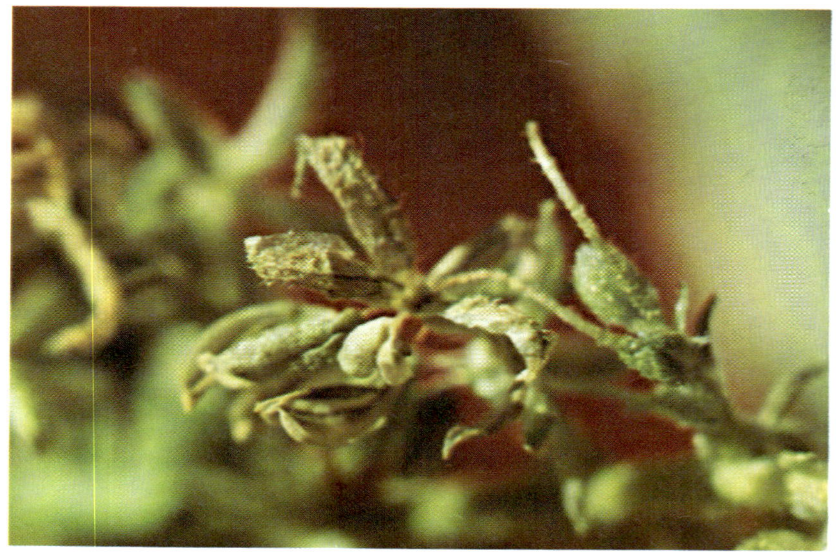

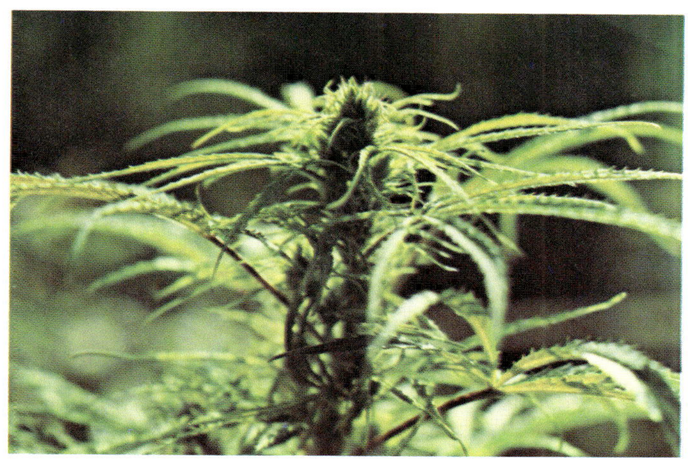

*tiny, green female flowers just beginning
to cluster on the tips of the branches
several weeks after the first flowers
showed at the nodes*

IT IS QUITE CLEAR that the time of planting is of prime significance in determining the male/female ratio. In winter, the sun is weak, the days are short and a majority of males will occur regardless of favorable weather. In spring, the sun returns and a more even ratio occurs. In the beginning of summer the earth receives the full force of the sun, and a majority of females is certain. Hermaphrodites and males are more abundant when plants are starved for sunlight or crowded upon one another. The plants must be given every opportunity to thrive and develop to their full potential.

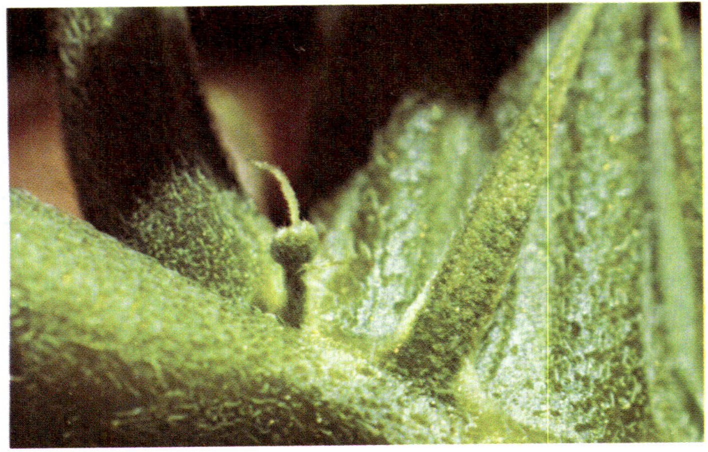

an early male sac with a protruding female pistil

THE CANNABIS is primarily determined to reproduce itself and sometimes it is impossible to deter this powerful mechanism. In sinsemilla, as the males are plucked, the females sense their condition and sometimes develop scattered male sacs in the colas in a desperate attempt at self-pollination. In some strains, even under ideal conditions, long before the males are pulled, sacs will occur at some of the nodes and later recede when the plant develops as a pure female.

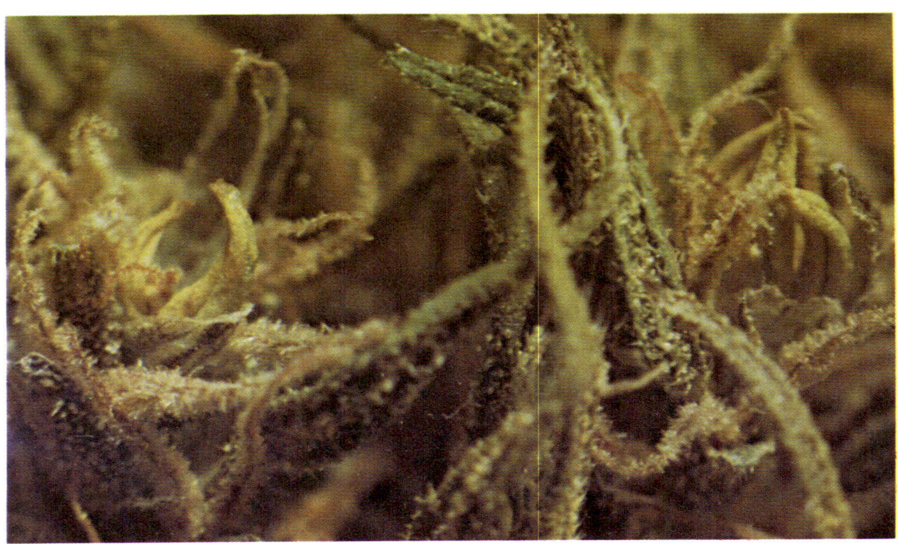

a dry female cluster with a few undeveloped, yellow male sacs

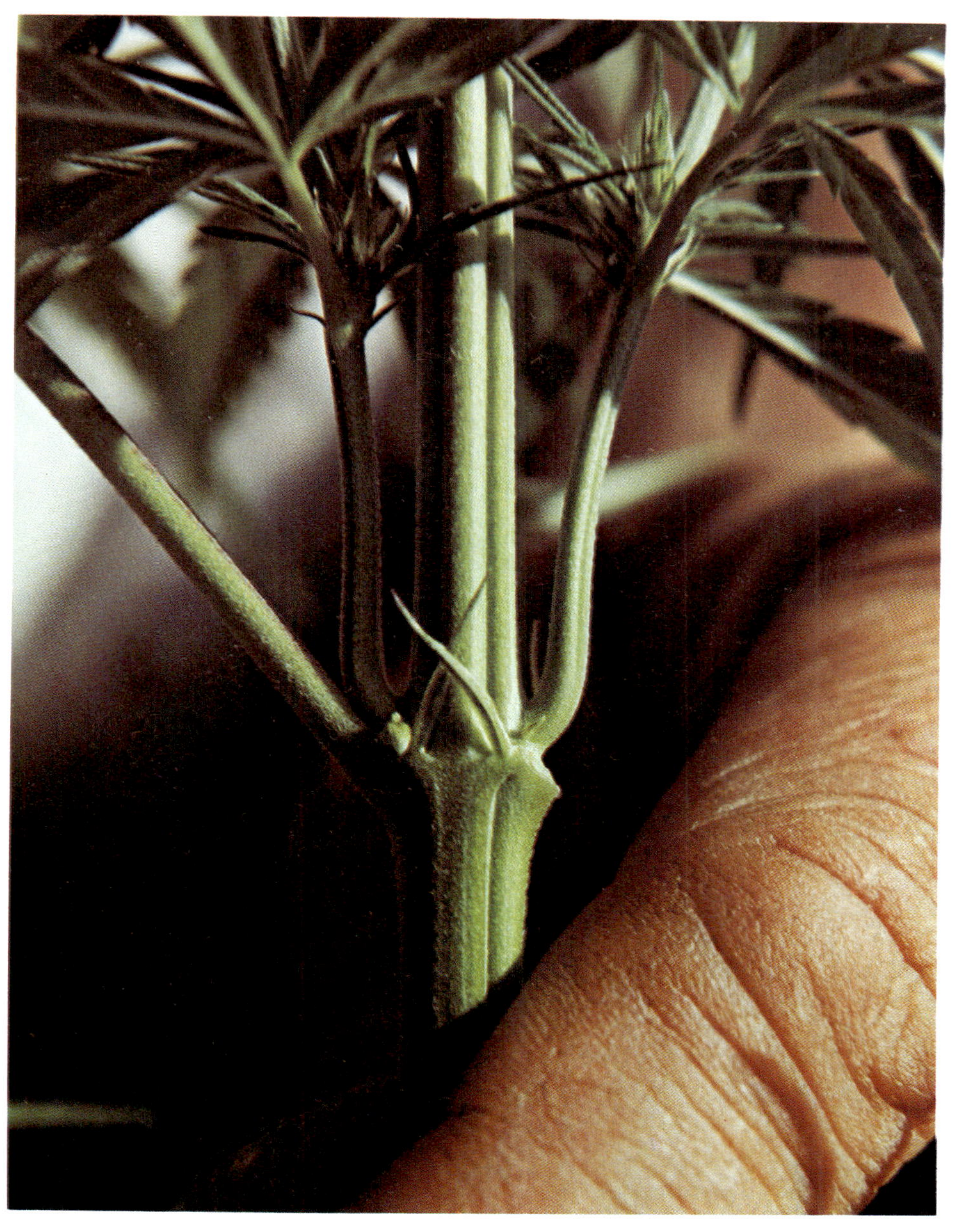

*this female had male sacs at some of the nodes—here the
male sac on the left is strangely more developed than
the female sheath on the right*

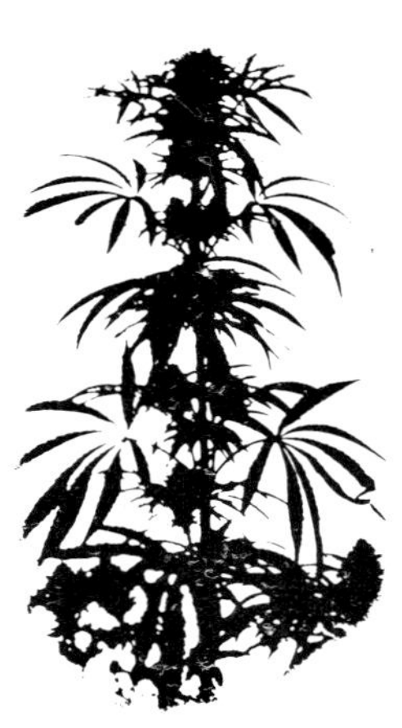

PART THREE

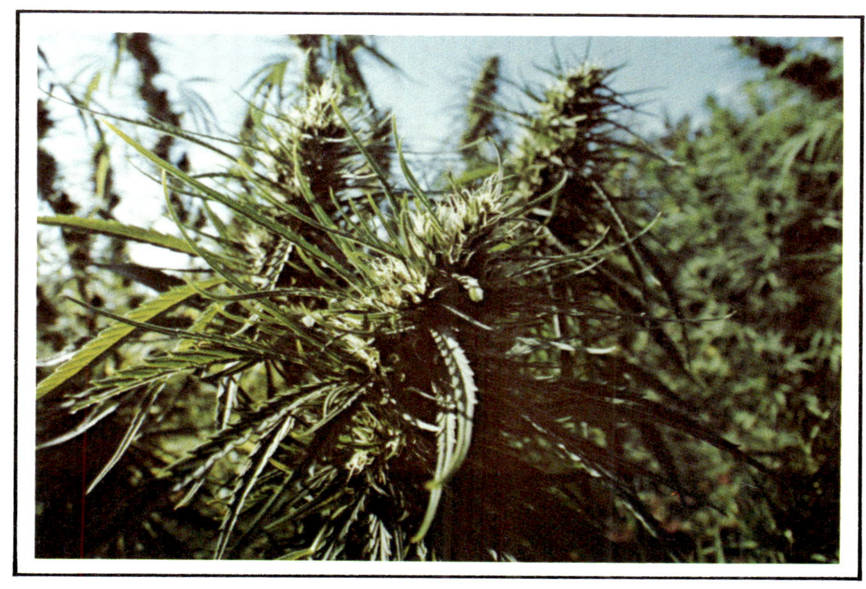

FLORESCENCE

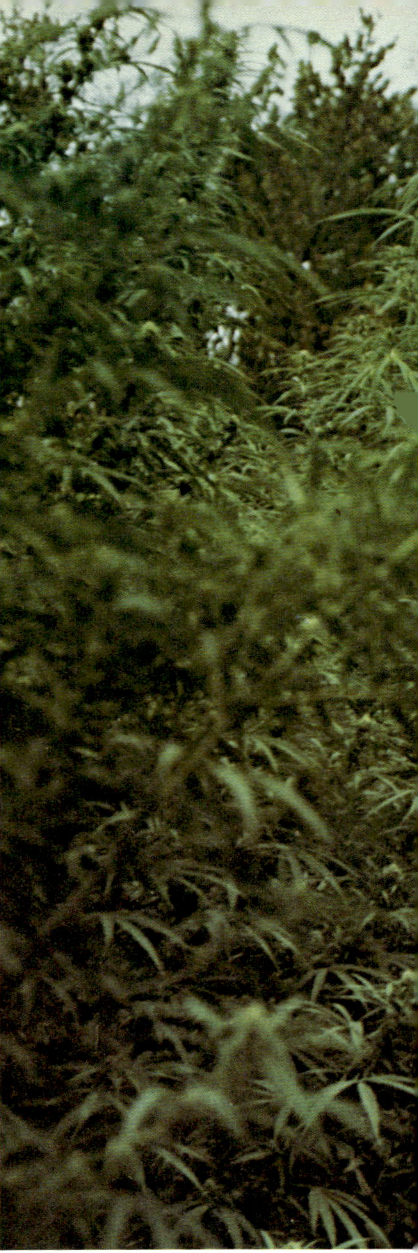

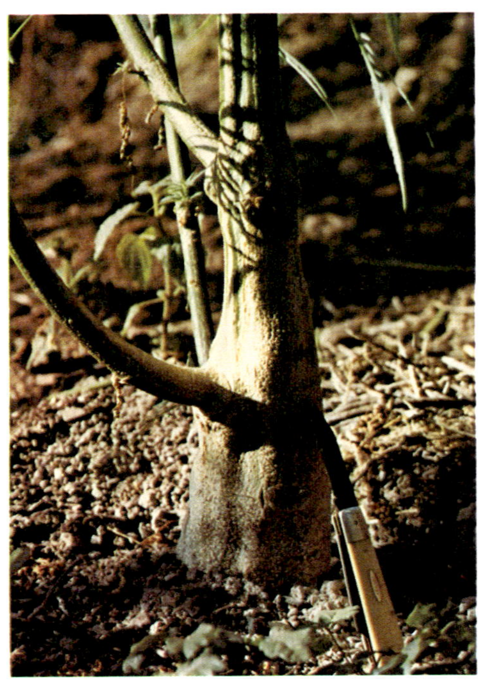

UNDER IDEAL CONDITIONS, the young hemp may grow more than an inch a day. Adolescent plants often double their size in six weeks at the onset of summer. Stalks swell as large as a man's arm and branch systems equal the growth of the main stalk. Some strains grow upward while others may spread more laterally. An extremely robust plant may reach twelve or fourteen feet and spread several feet across. To attain full potential, strict spacing must be kept between the plants. Three feet is minimum but five is better if the soil is rich and the climate is mellow. The size of the plant and the colas reflect the health of the organism but do not necessarily indicate the quality of the smoke obtained from the flowers.

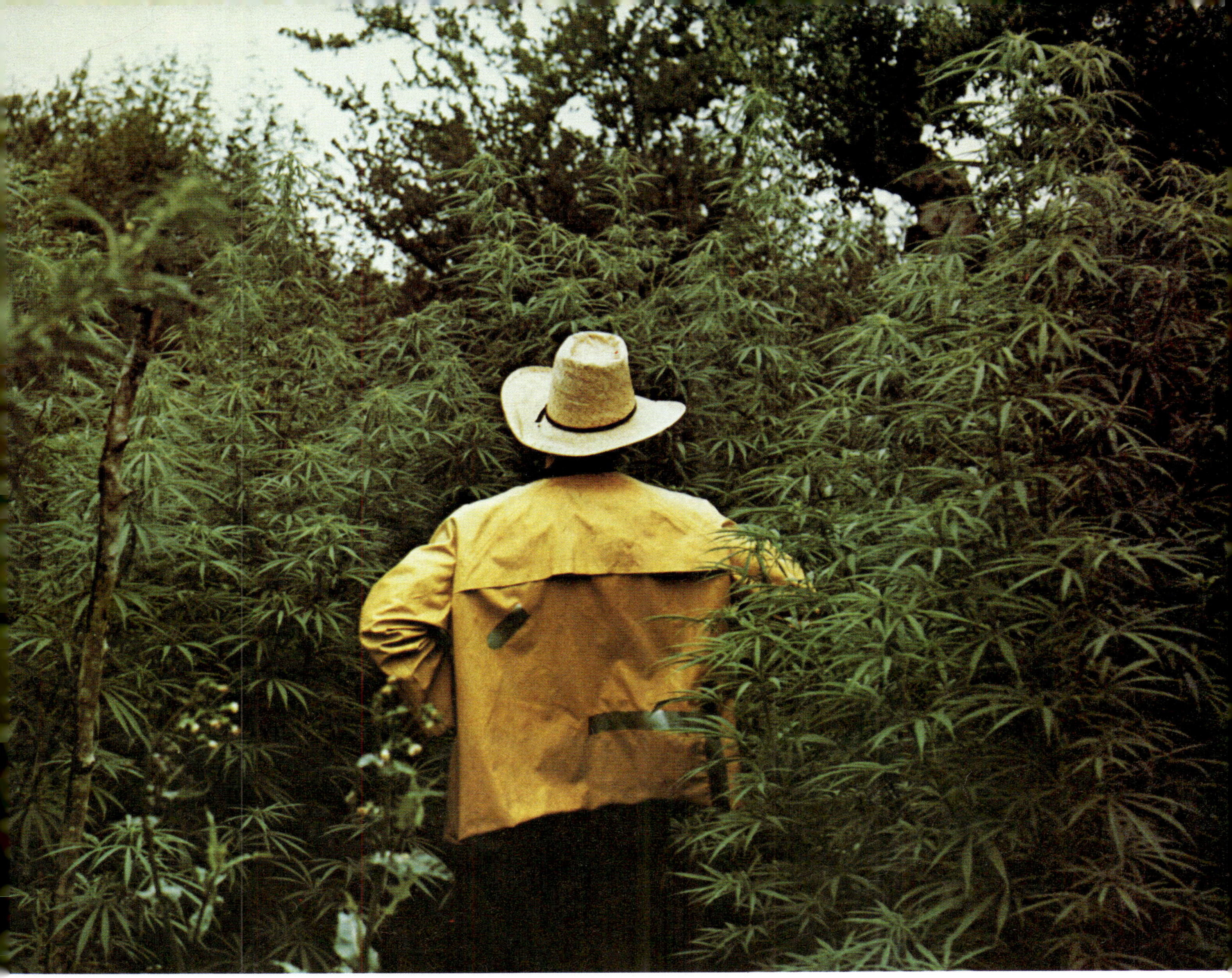

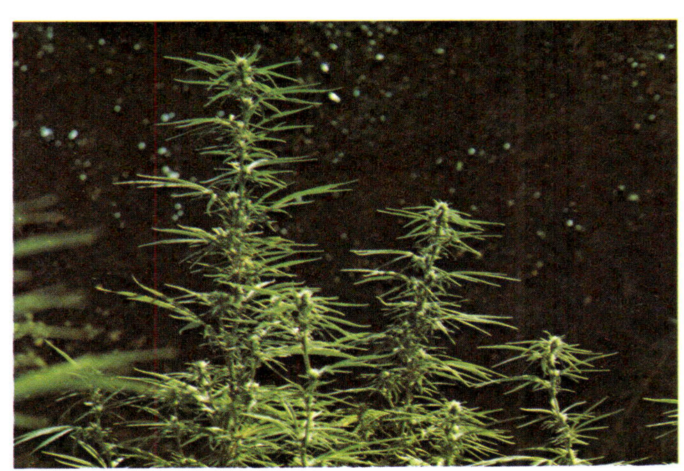

at first the flowering tips are small
and translucent green

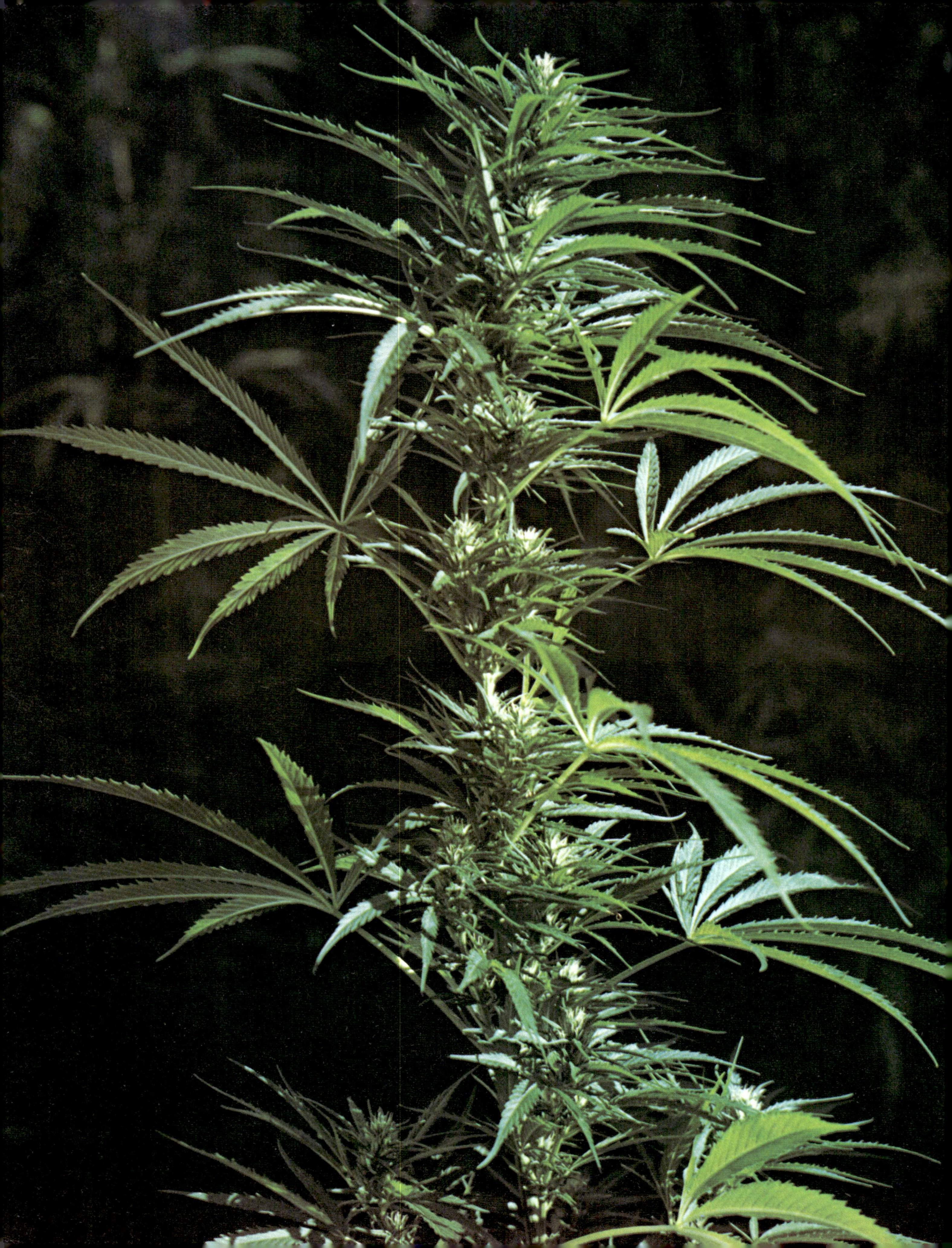

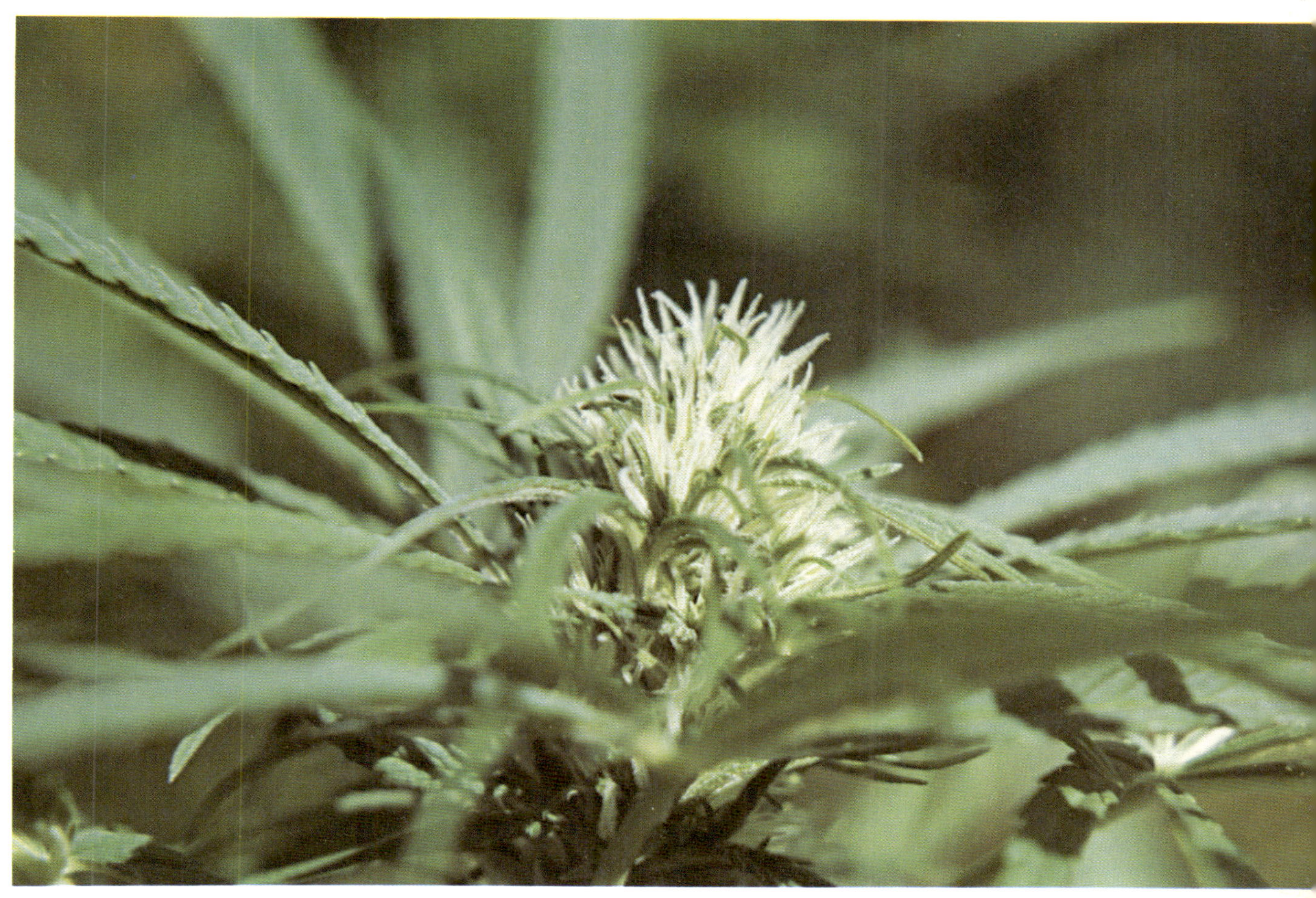

a young budding female, her feathery clusters just beginning to swell

IN LATE SUMMER, growth is at its peak and the plants reach their maximum size. At first the flower clusters grow slowly but now they are beginning to swell noticeably. As the plant begins its rush to bloom, the intense upward growth slows and finally ceases altogether. As the sexual energies of the plant come to maturity, the rhythm of the dance intensifies. The days shorten as the sun fades to the south. The organism is tuned to a single objective: regeneration of the species—seed production.

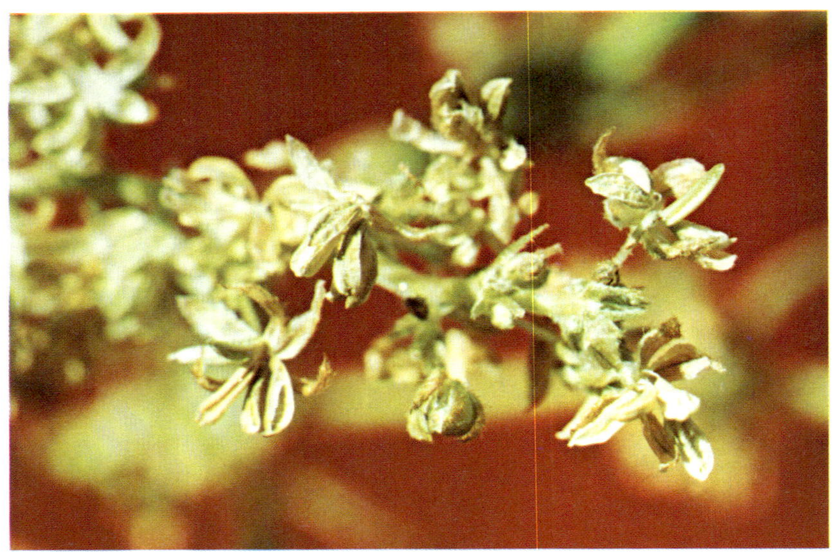

*in seeded hemp the males release clouds of pollen (above)
which create thousands of seeds in the female (below)*

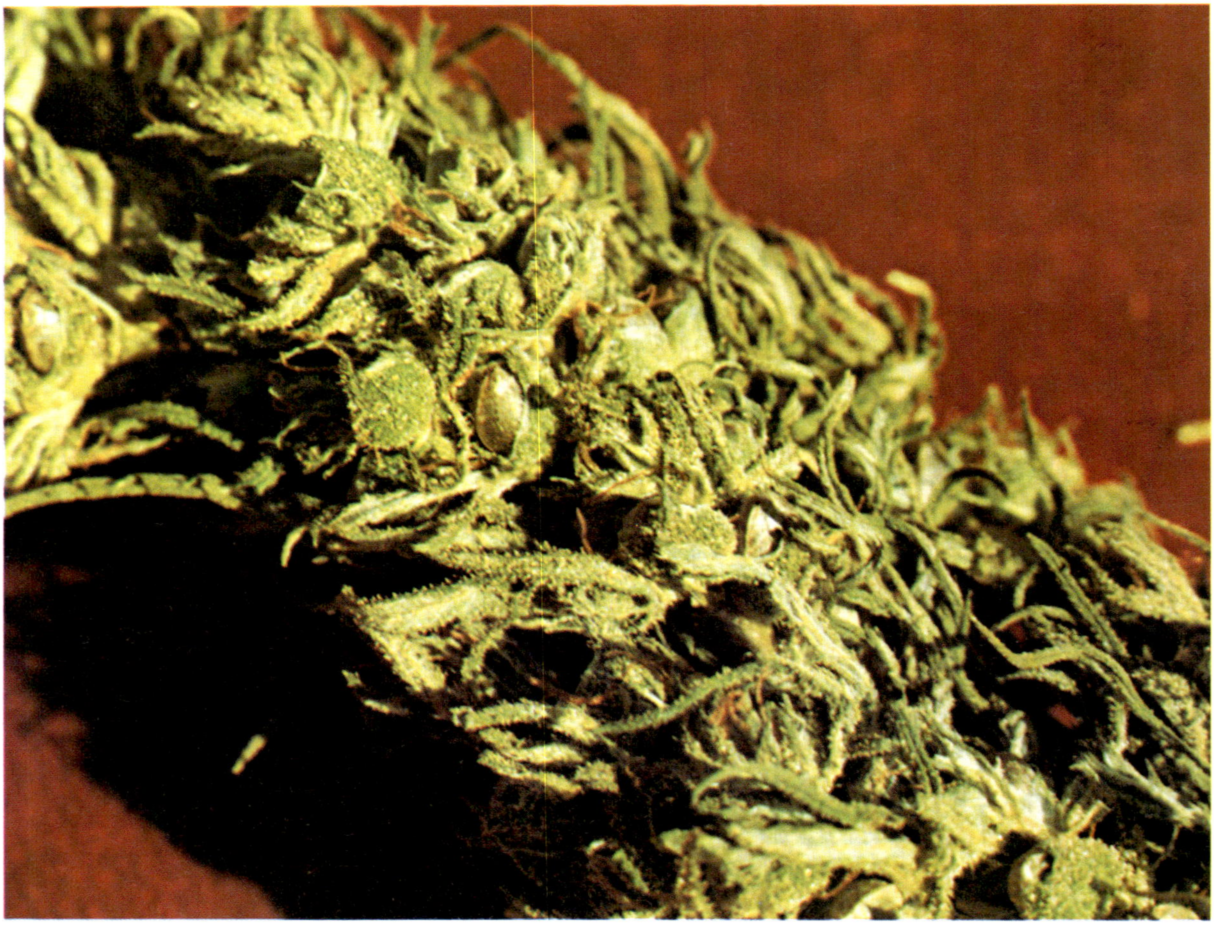

ALLOWED TO FOLLOW its natural cycle, the uncultivated cannabis must produce enormous quantities of seed to assure the survival of sufficient offspring. Clouds of pollen create thousands of seeds from which only a small portion survive. Birds and rodents eat their share and many rot in the dampness or fall upon barren soil. From handfuls of seed, perhaps a few plants live to complete another cycle. Like most plants, the hemp reproduces itself by sheer mass of pollen and seed. It is this primal reproductive energy which is gently altered to create sinsemilla.

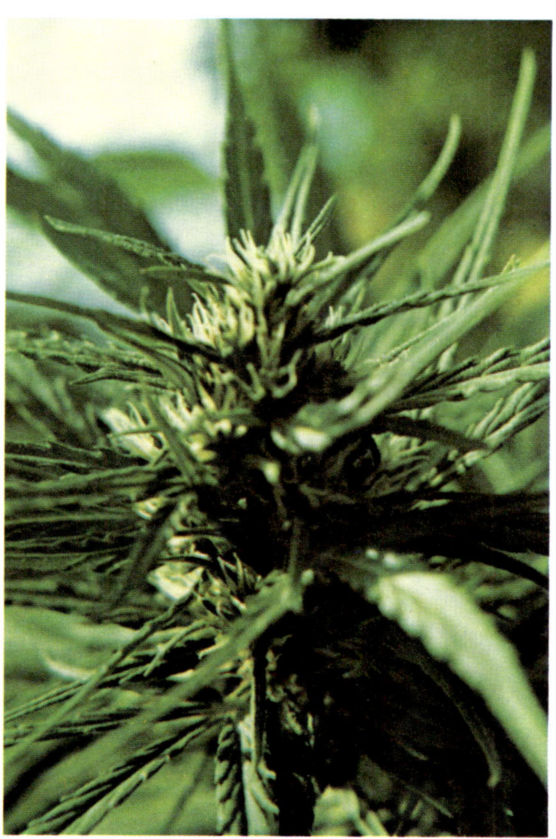

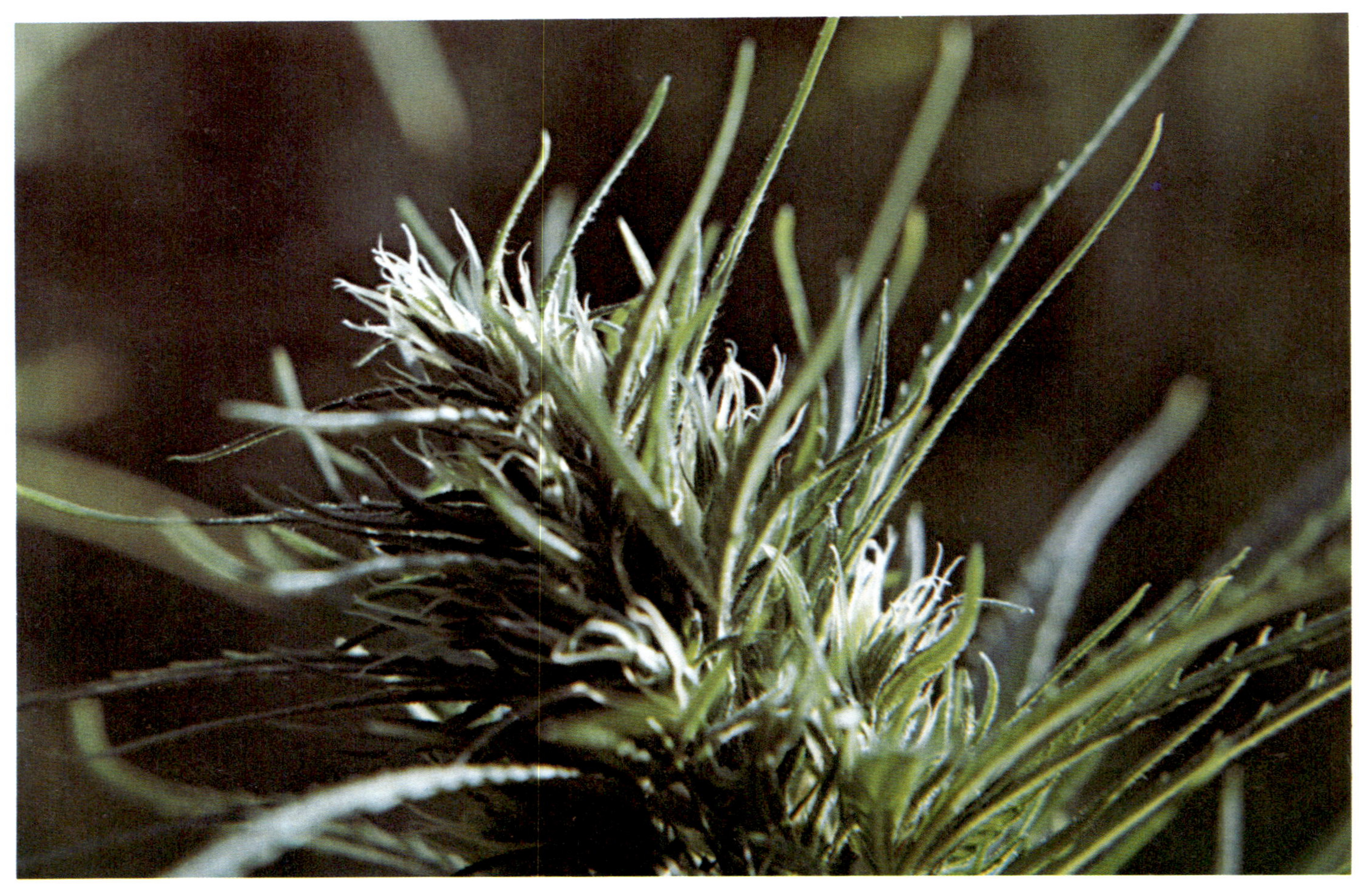

HERE LIES THE BASIC DIFFERENCE between the seeded
and unseeded varieties of the cannabis. In pollinated plants, as the
flowers appear, the pistils receive the male dust and transmit the
energy to the ovaries in the pods below. After fertilization, the
pistils shrivel and die. For a period of days the bloom is intense
but there is no single unified bloom. For several weeks the cycle
is repeated again and again in each plant. As the flower dies, the
seed is born. If the plants are harvested when the seeds are mature,
the flowers are long gone. Their sweetness is short-lived.

IN SINSEMILLA the rhythm is different. The unpollinated plant continues to amass fresh blossoms for many weeks and the blossoms are not spoiled by pollen. The clusters remain delicate and fragrant until the peak of florescence, when the energy of the whole plant reaches maturity. All the flowers are sweet and ripe, and no potency has been lost to seed. The sweetness expresses the clarity of the smoke.

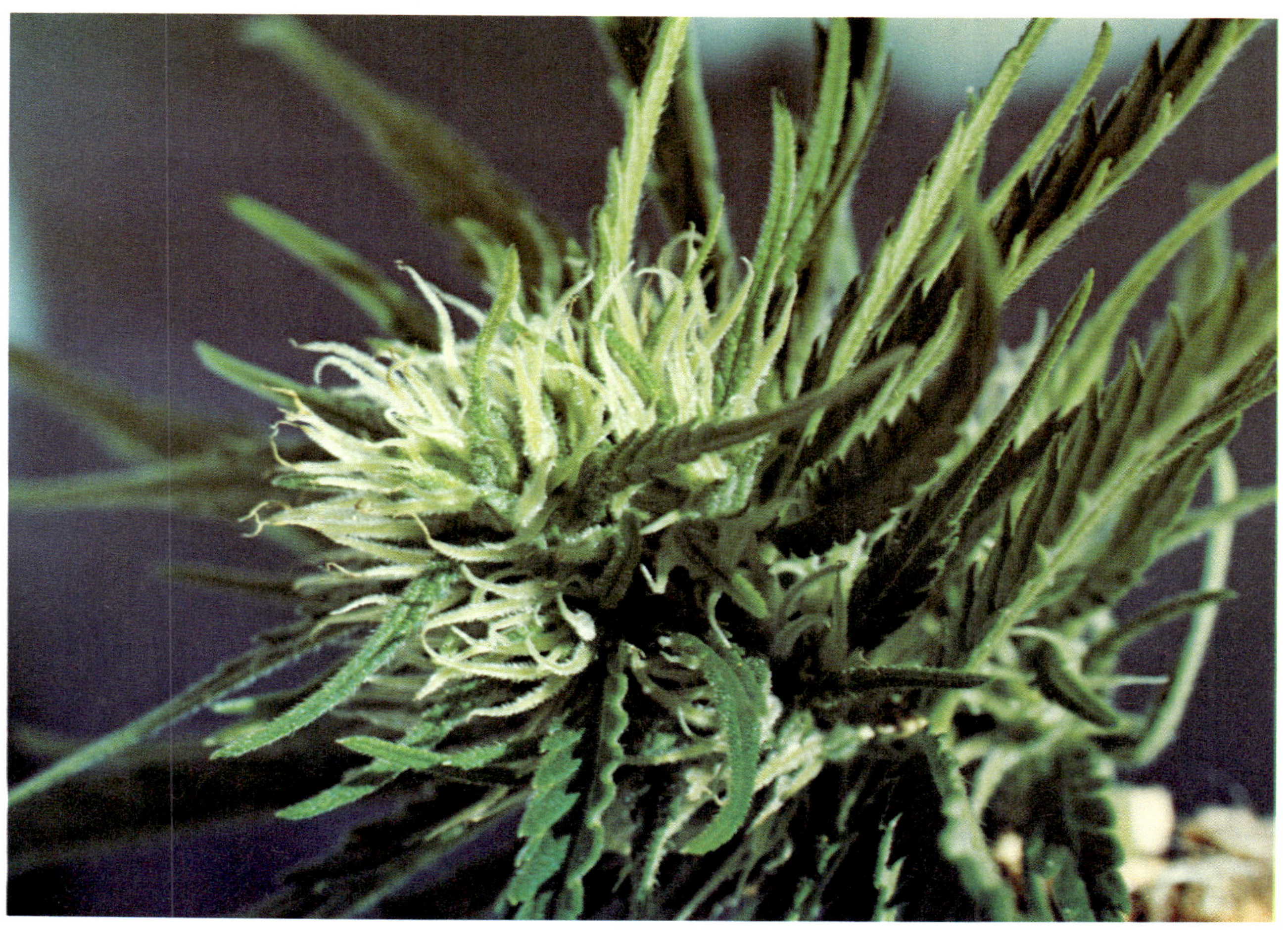

dense clusters of pistils still young and growing

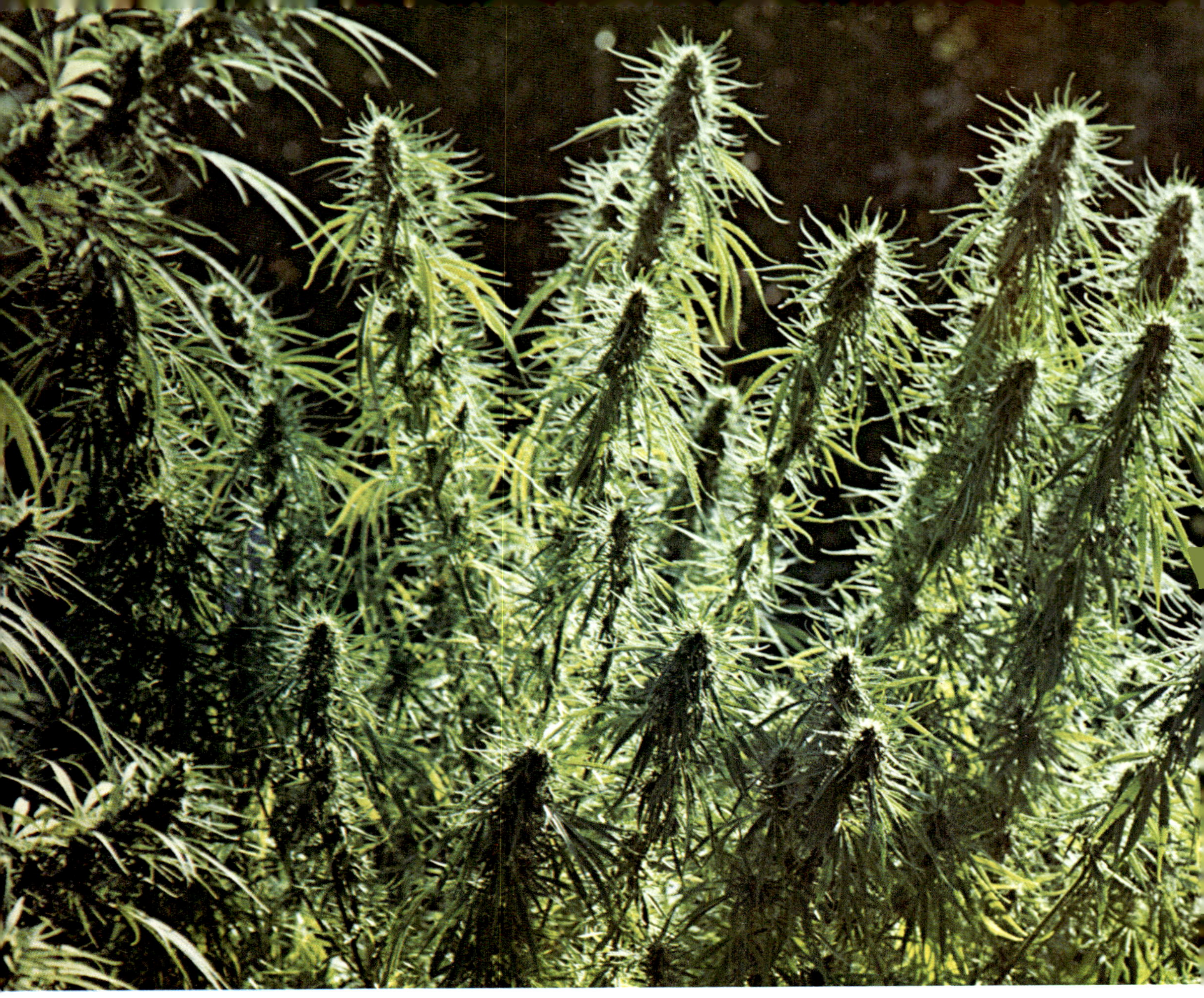

electric sinsemilla colas swelling with energy

IMAGINE THE SWELLING ENERGY of the flowering plant, each day amassing more fresh blossoms awaiting pollination. The flowers crowd in upon one another in dense clusters. The virgin blossoms swell with sexual energy eager for consummation. But the breeze brings no pollen and the rhythm continues to intensify.

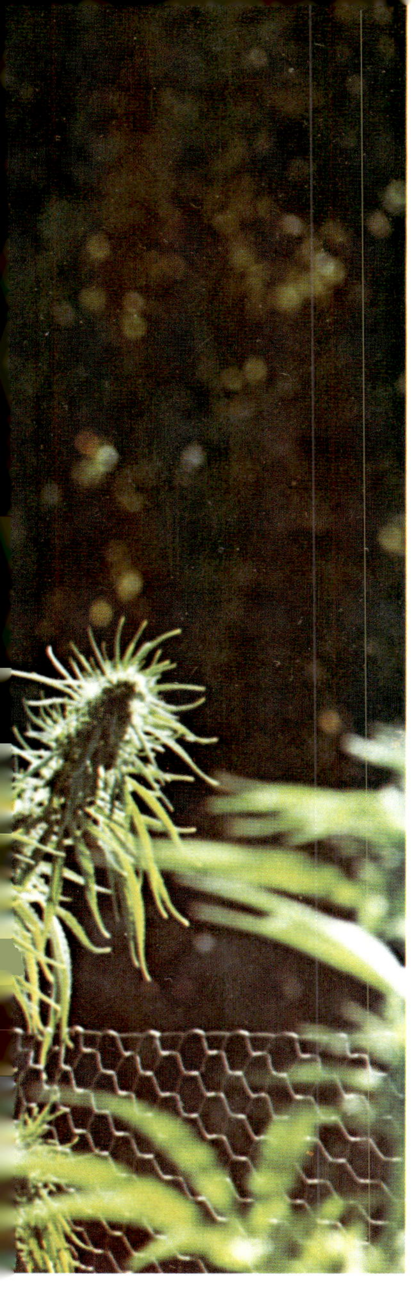

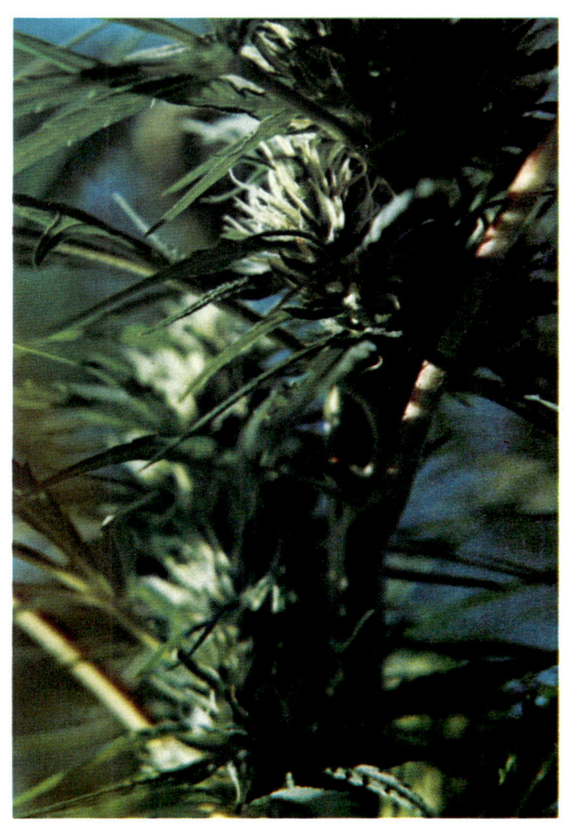

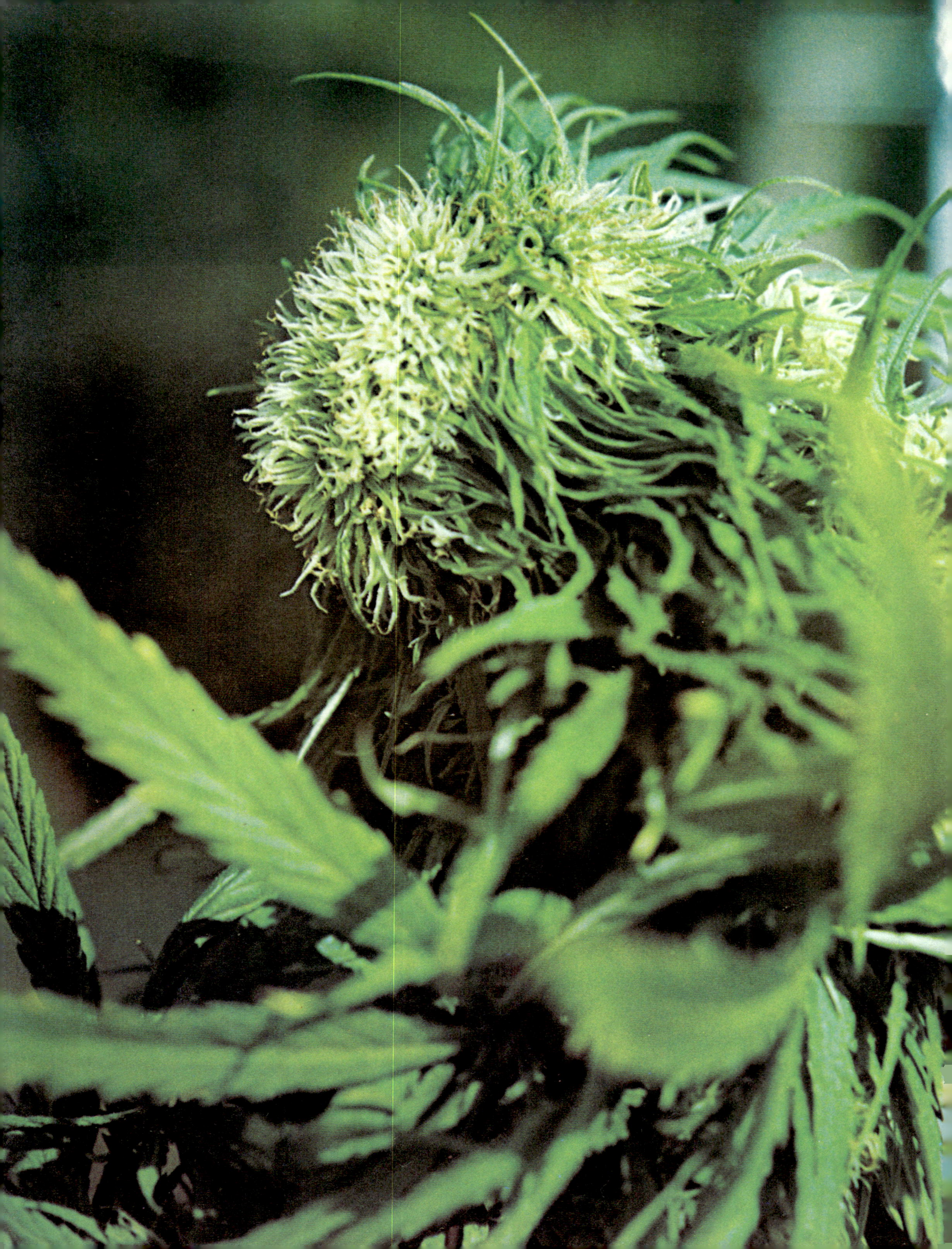

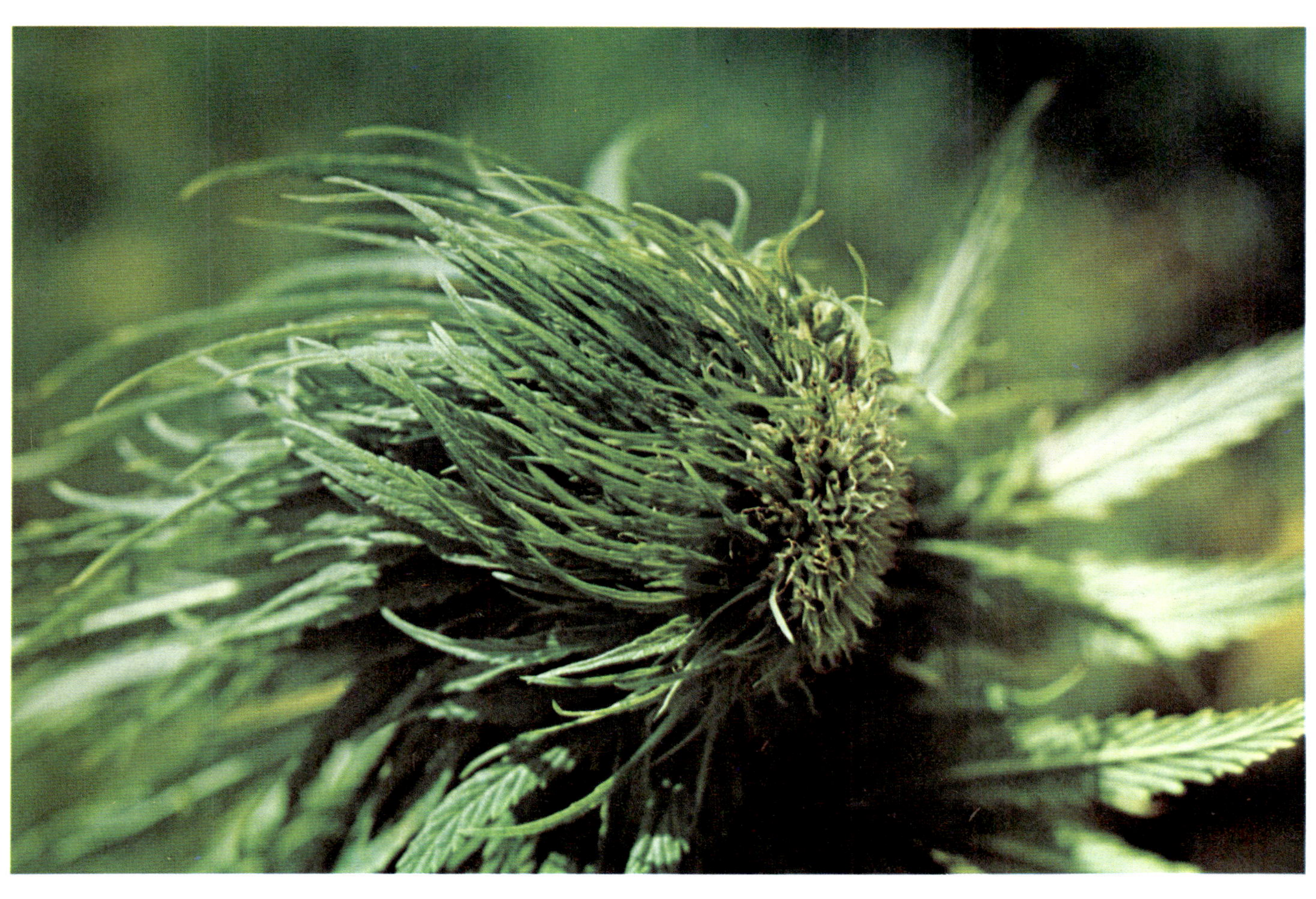

*This is a strange and amazing formation which occasionally occurs in the tip of a branch —
the stem flattens and the cluster bends in a hook. The pistils become incredibly dense
and leave no room for leaf*

FOR SEVERAL WEEKS, the tips of the clusters fill out with more and more pistils. The older blossoms swell, remaining green and translucent. As the last pistils come into the tips, the clusters turn pure white. The pods swell and the resinous coating thickens. The true sweetness of the flowers comes forth and becomes so strong it is almost too much to bear. This is a time of waiting and watching and breathing in the scent of the blossoms. Within a few days the seedless clusters will be at the height of their potency.

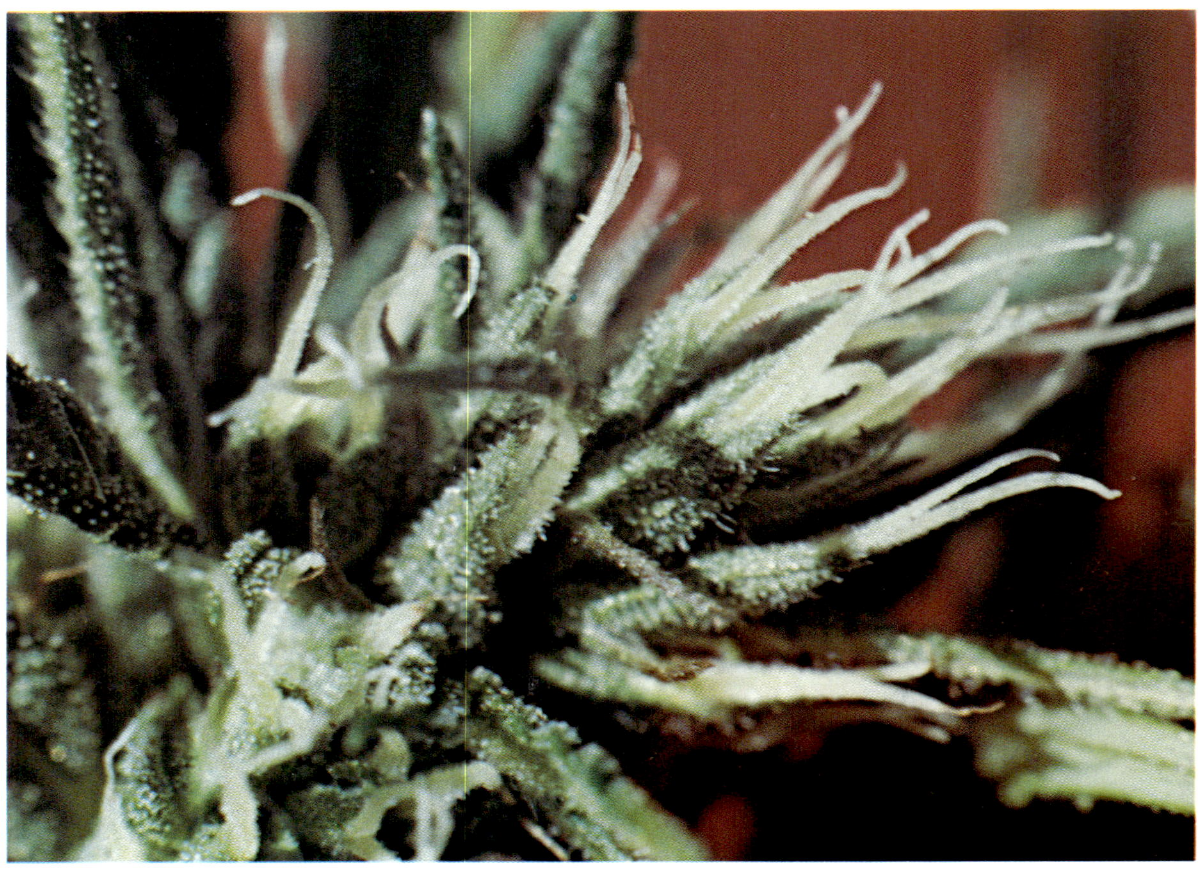

A magnified view of the opposite photo—long, sinuous pistils are reaching out for pollen. The empty seed covers are not quite fully swollen, but ripeness is near.

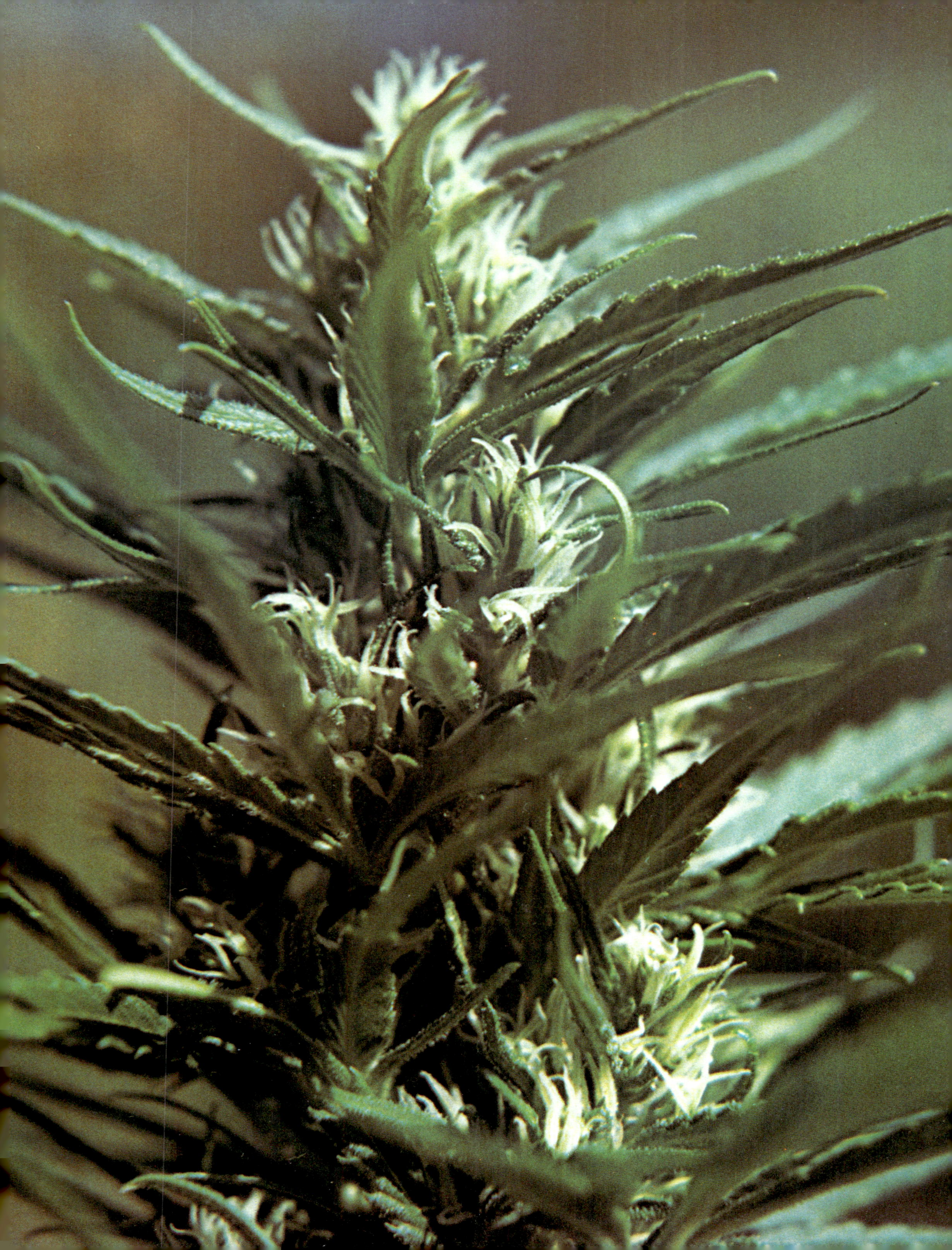

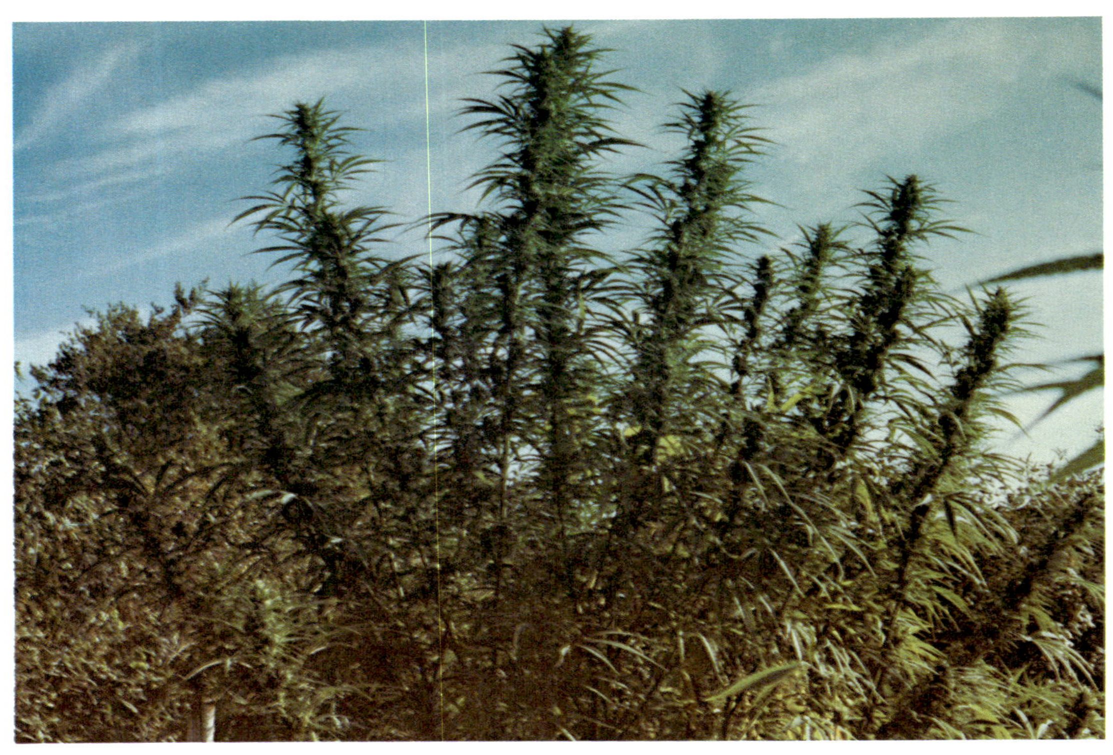

the plant (above), the colas (below) and the flowers (opposite)

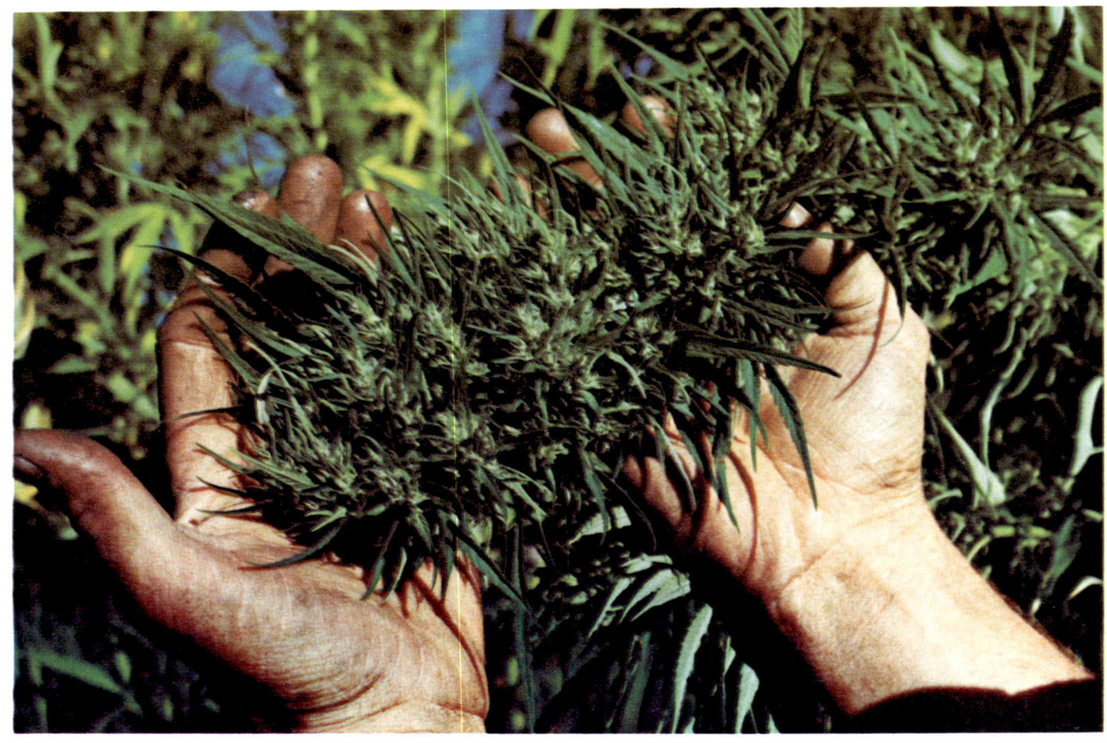

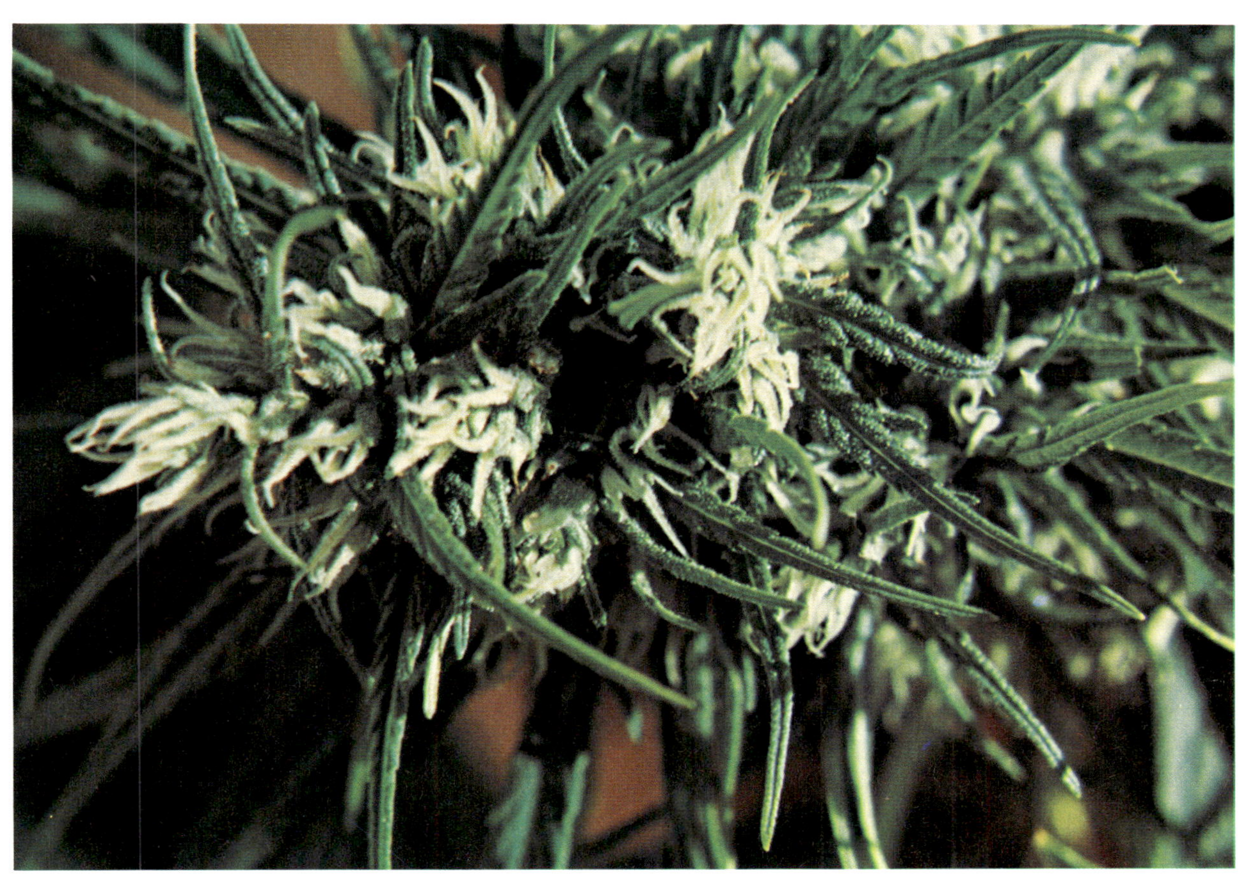

pistils, snow white just before harvest

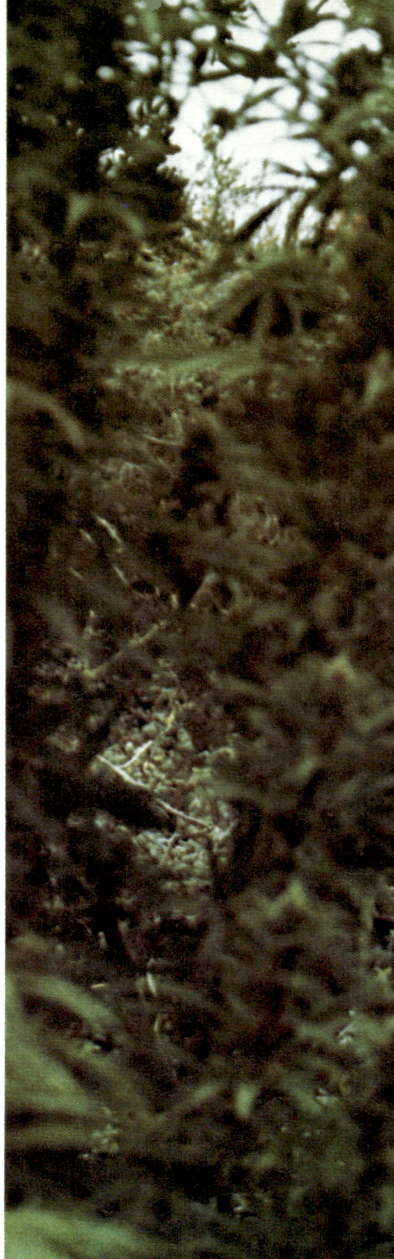

*The flower clusters swell to tremendous size
and glisten white in the tips of the branches.
The larger fan leaves often yellow and fall
to the ground as the flowers ripen.*

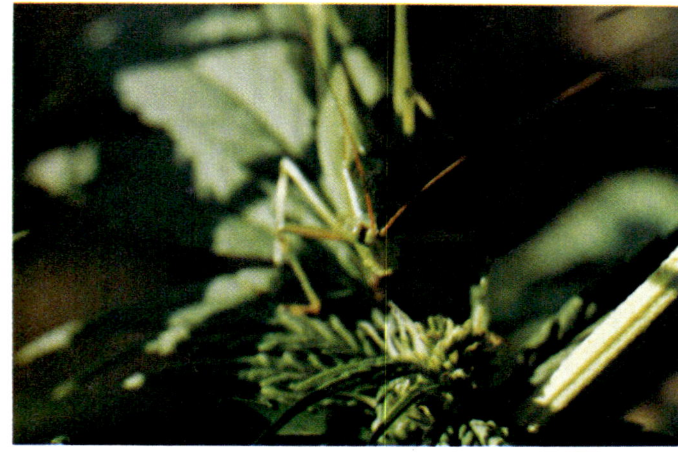

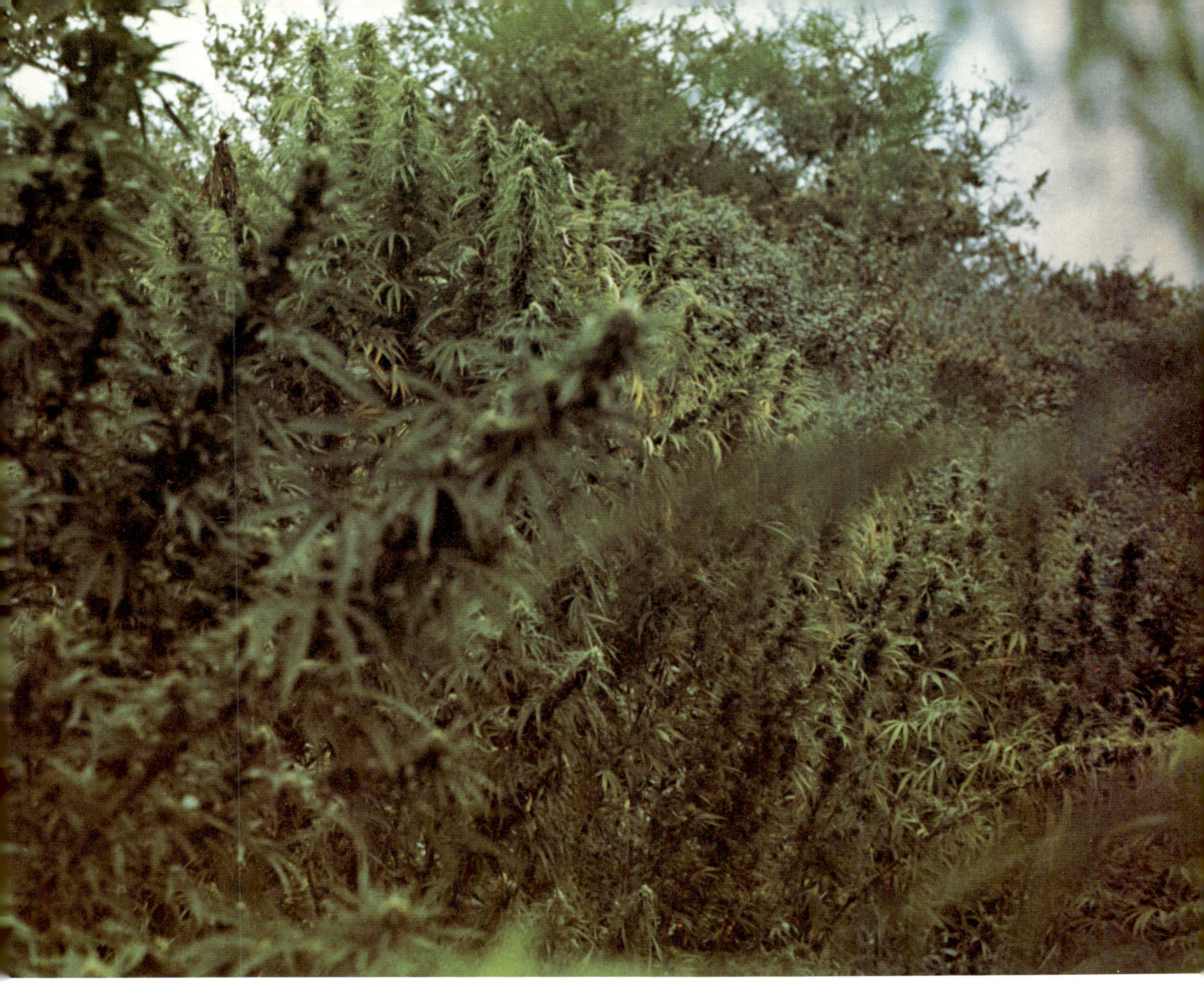

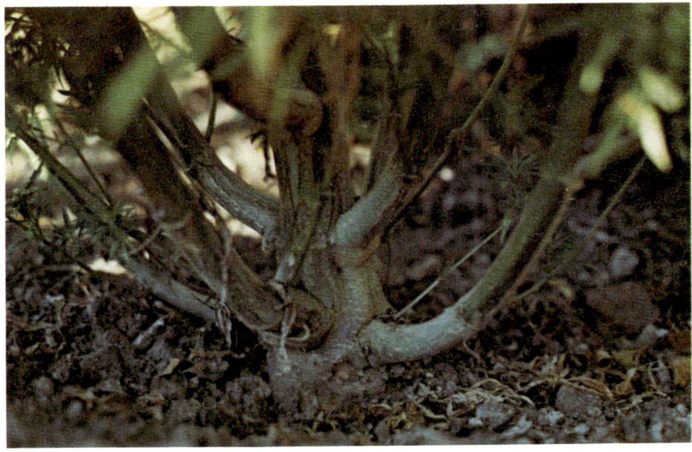

*the green plant above ground has its
corresponding growth below*

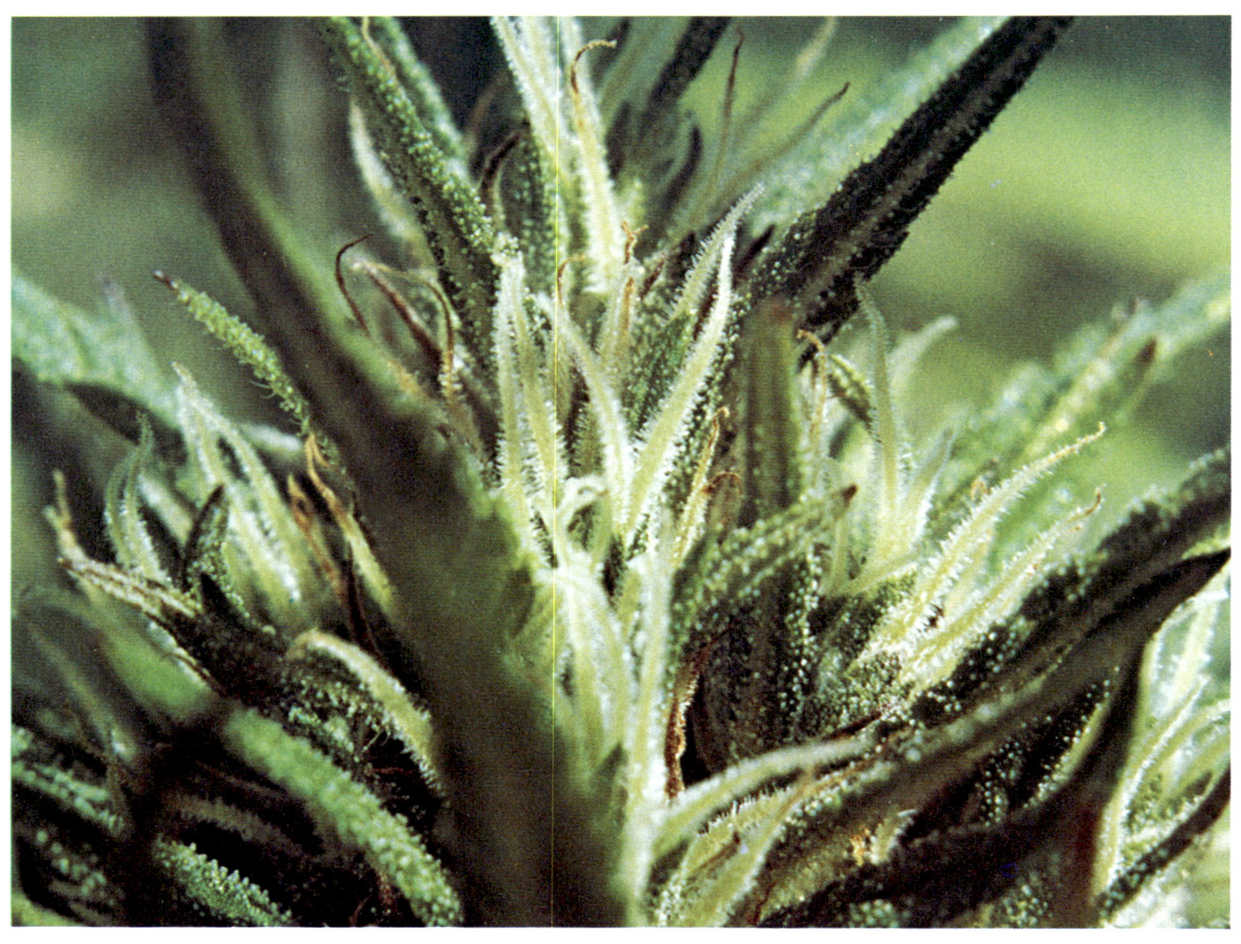

the peak of florescence: harvest

FINALLY THE SEEDLESS PLANT reaches the height of bloom. Florescence is complete and the plant has no more to give. The pistils are fresh and receptive, still awaiting pollination. Their whiteness turns to rich cream, almost yellow. Soon the pistils begin to curl in upon themselves, bending under the weight of their own fullness. The virgin blossoms exude their sweetness as if to coax the male to come near and taste their rare sinsemilla beauty. Resin sparkles everywhere like fine sugar coating. The moment is ripe for harvest. The energies of the flowers are climaxing.

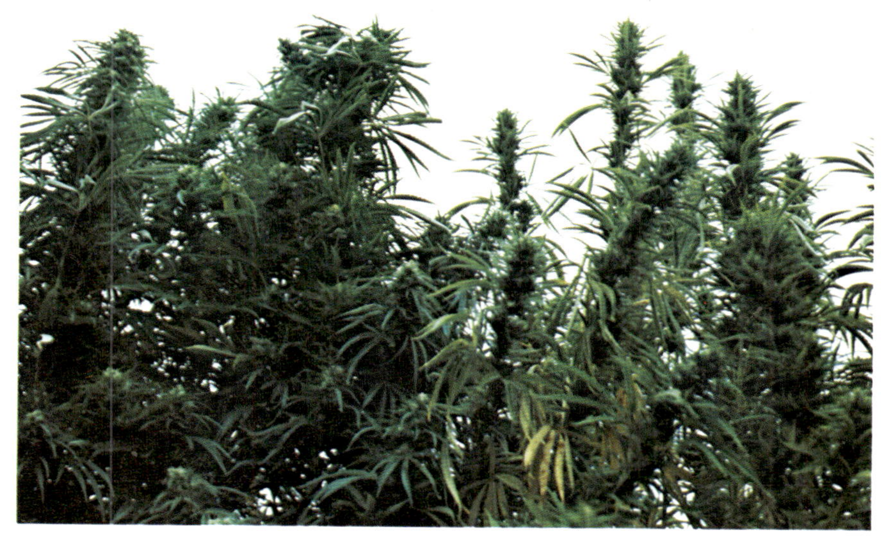

colas shoot up into the air like fat bottle brushes

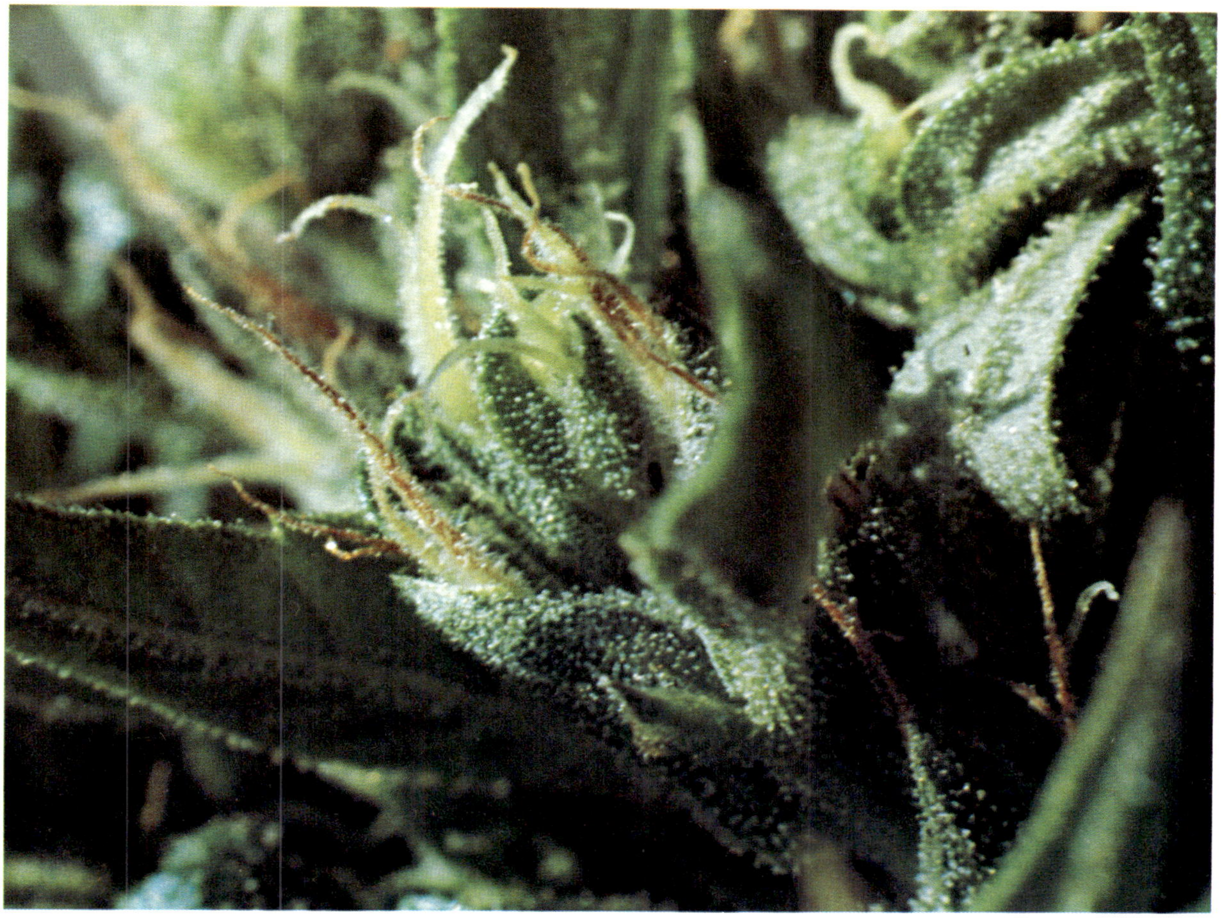

slight deterioration in the hairs and fully ripe, empty pods

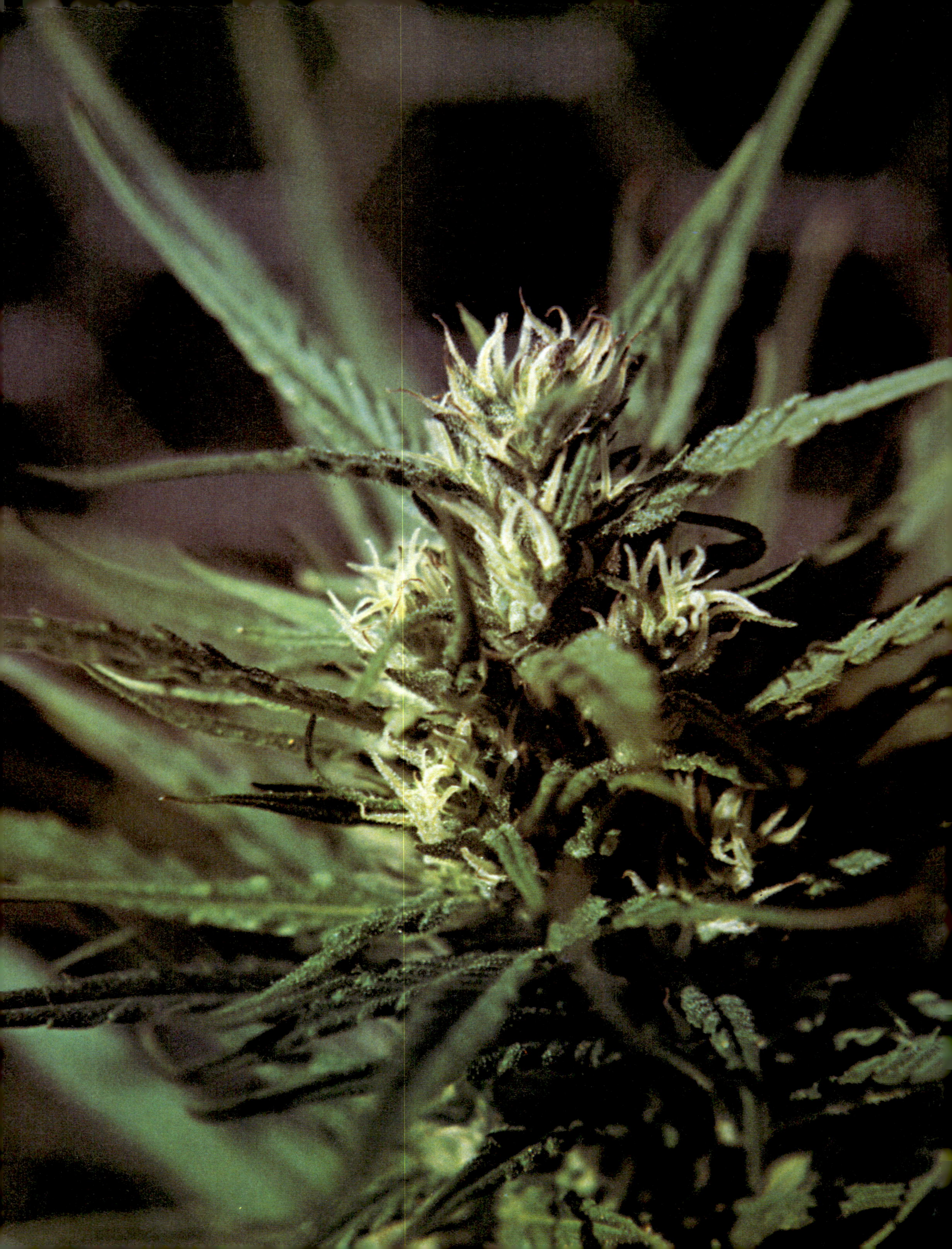

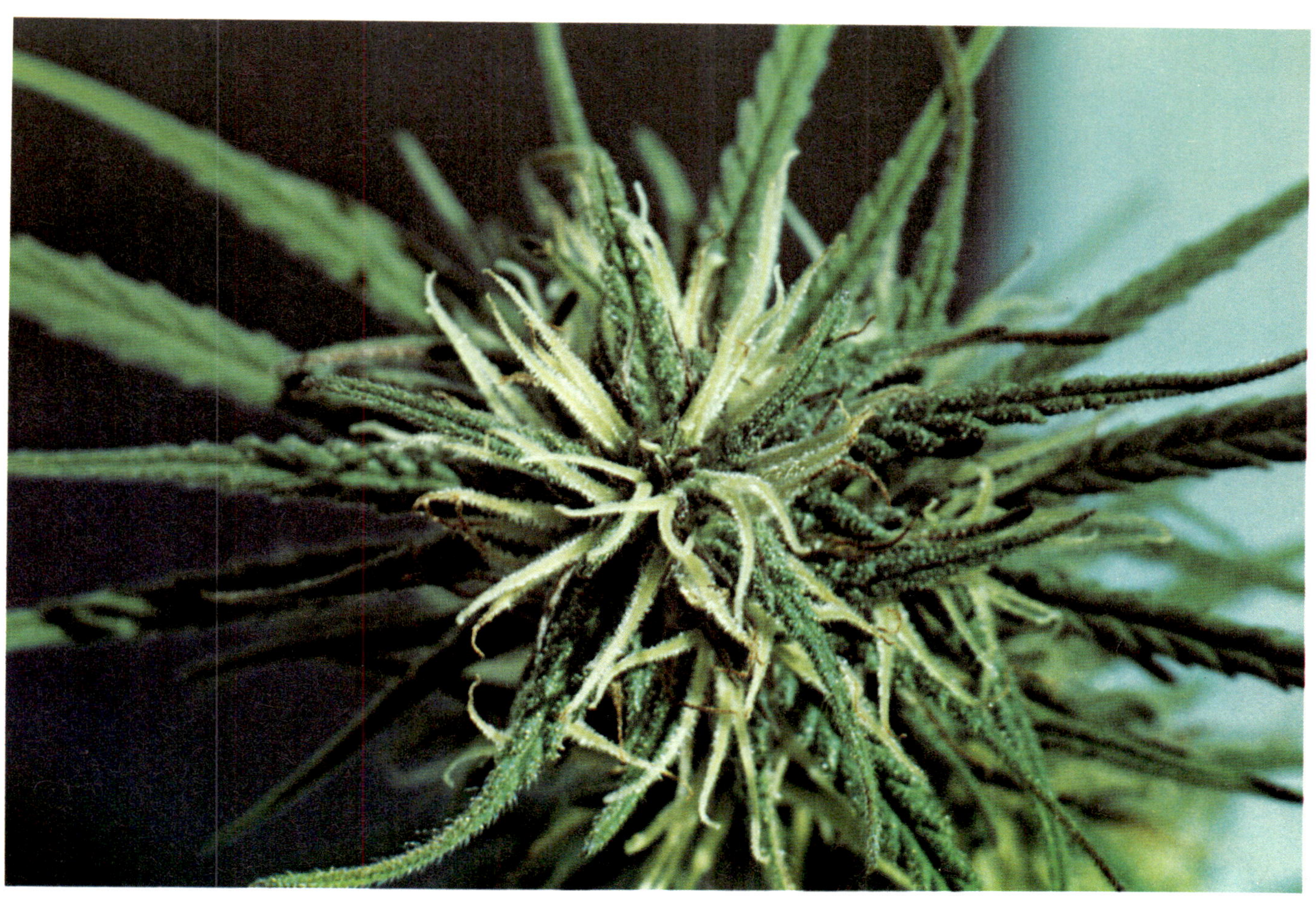

*a faint tinge of purple has shown in these tips as they are ready for harvest—
the pistils are full and some have browned from rain*

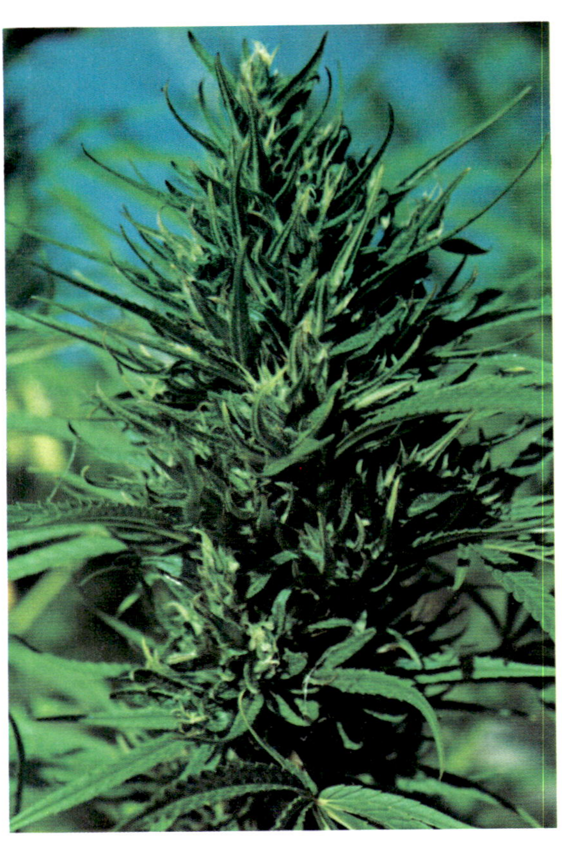

four shots of a cola at harvest: the whole cluster (above),
the lower flowers in the cluster (below) are extremely
swollen and show signs of age, while the flowers in the tips
(opposite) are still perfectly fresh

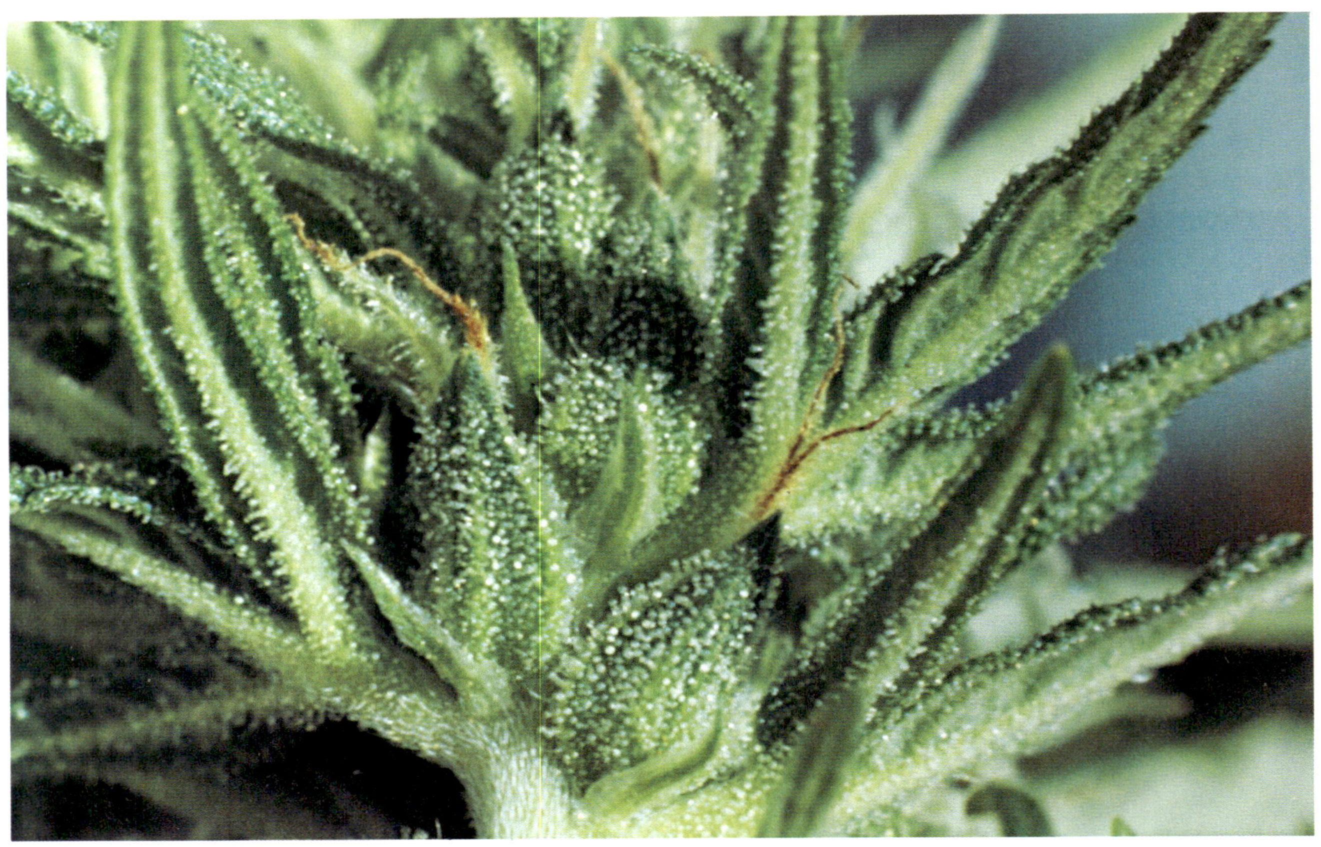

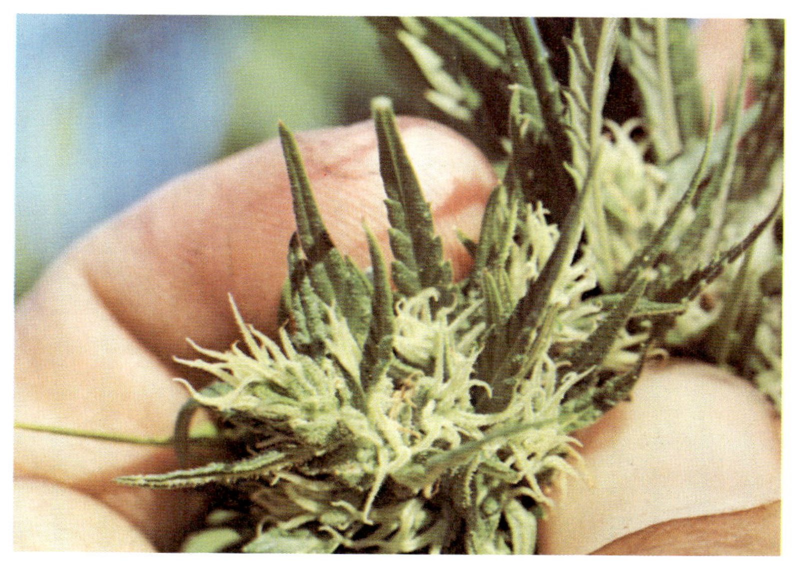

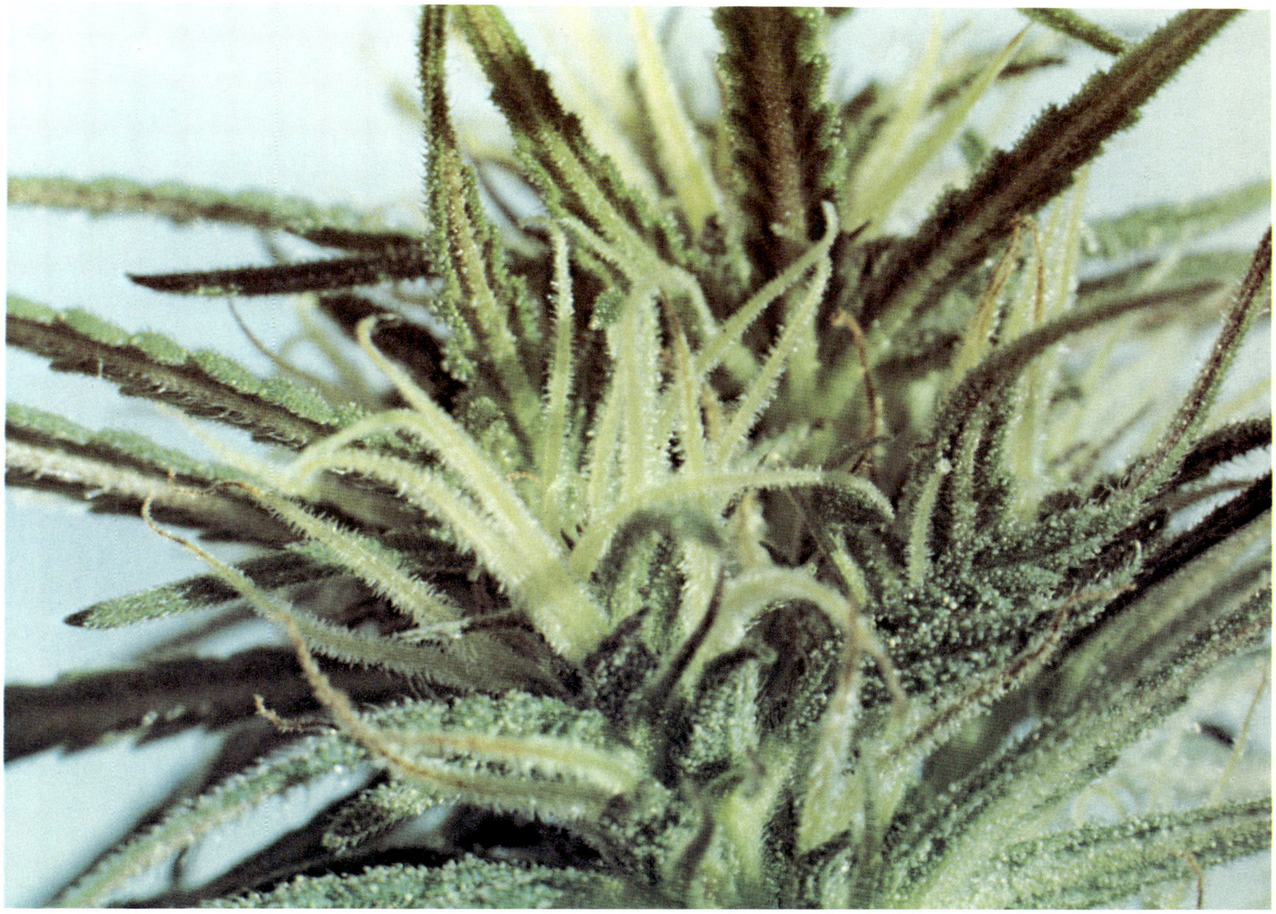

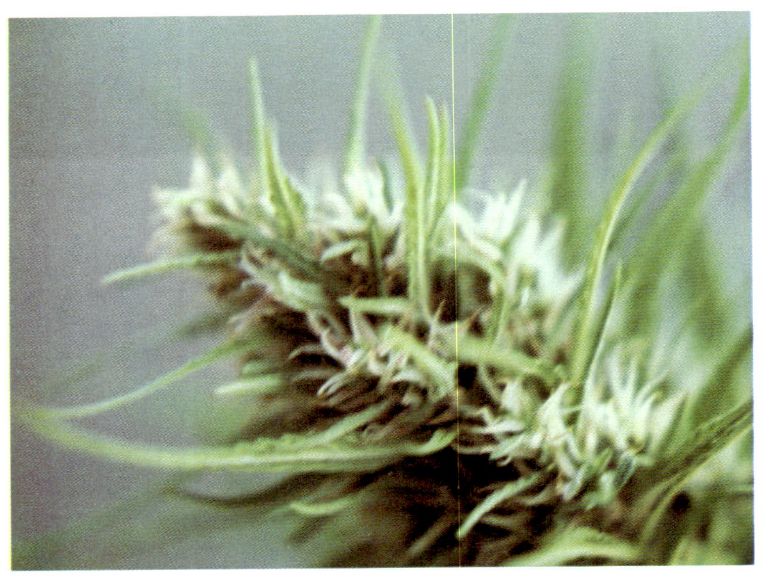

*some plants will show red or magenta in the pistils at maturity—
this is largely related to soil variation*

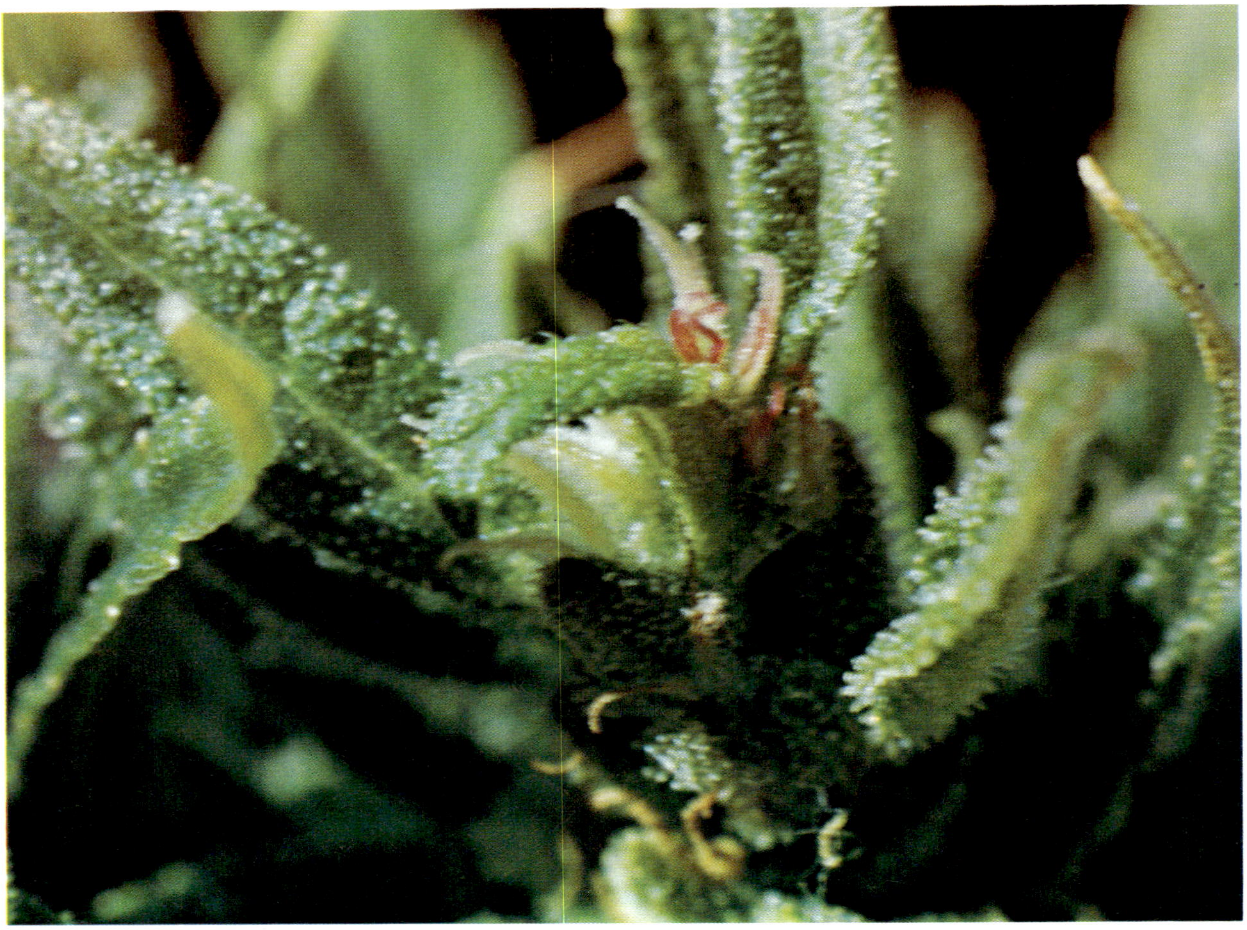

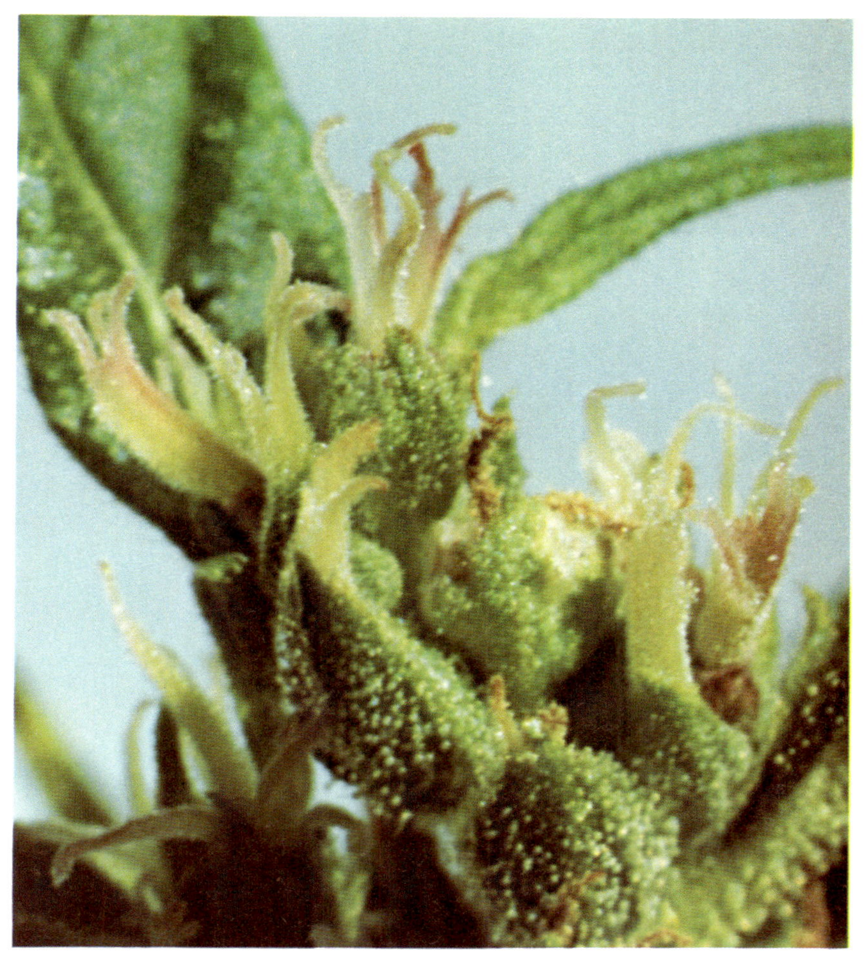

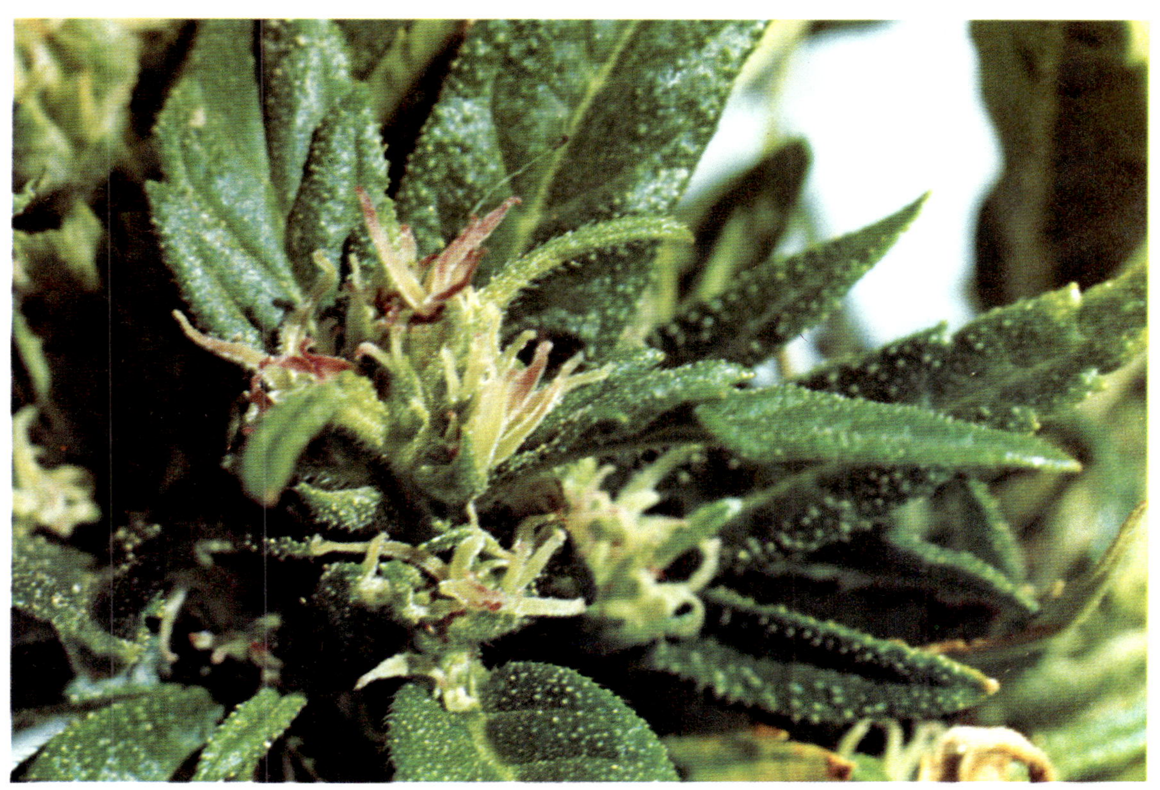

THE FLOWERS RETAIN their freshness for a few days, but they soon begin to deteriorate. The pistils in the tips dry and begin to wither away, the soft whiteness turning to brown. Sinsemilla florescence passes and the colas grow fat with age.

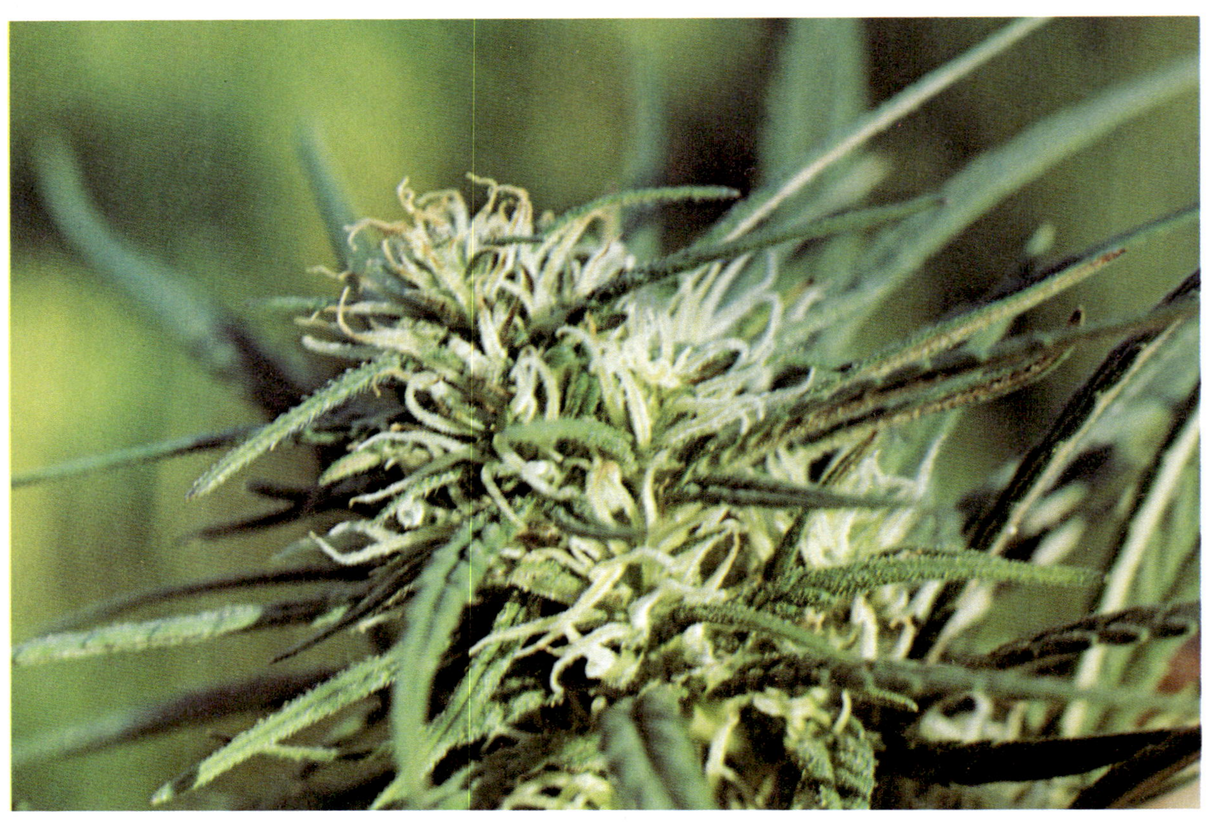

*the pistils have begun to curl in upon themselves like white worms—
the tips are browning and beginning to die*

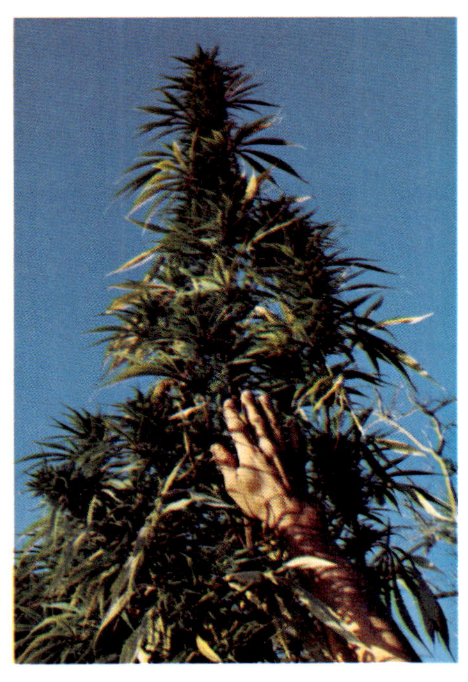

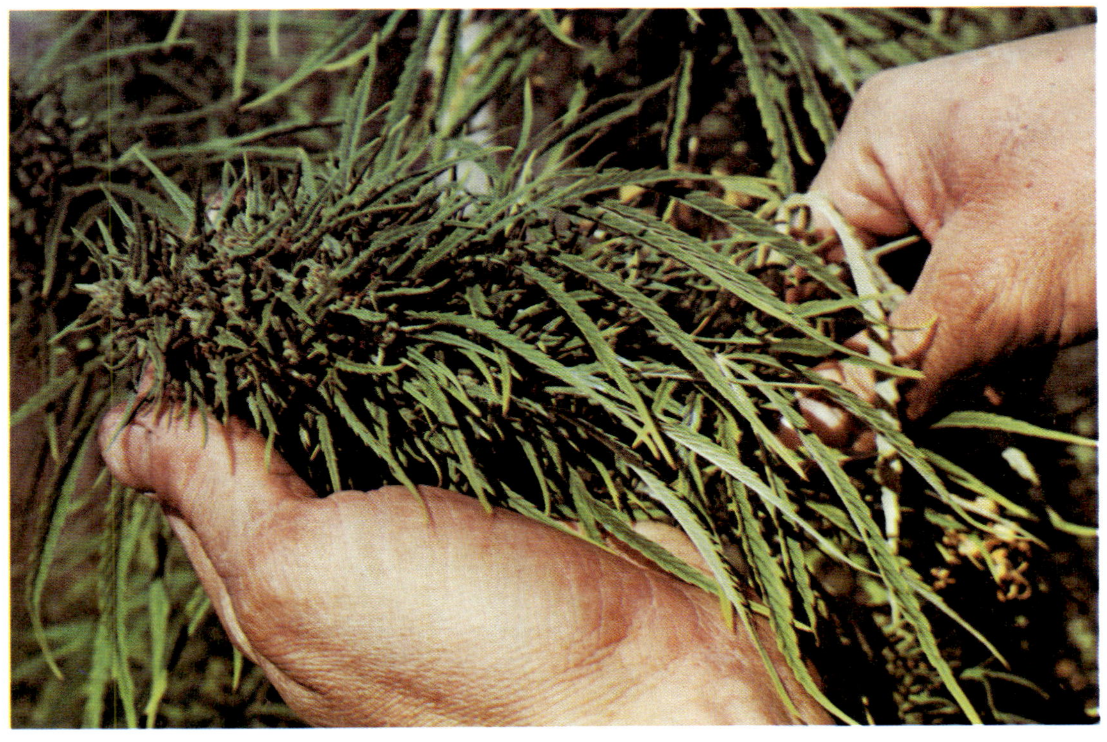

*about a week later, the whiteness is gone and the leaves have begun
to swell with age—the fine edge of the fresh flowers has been lost*

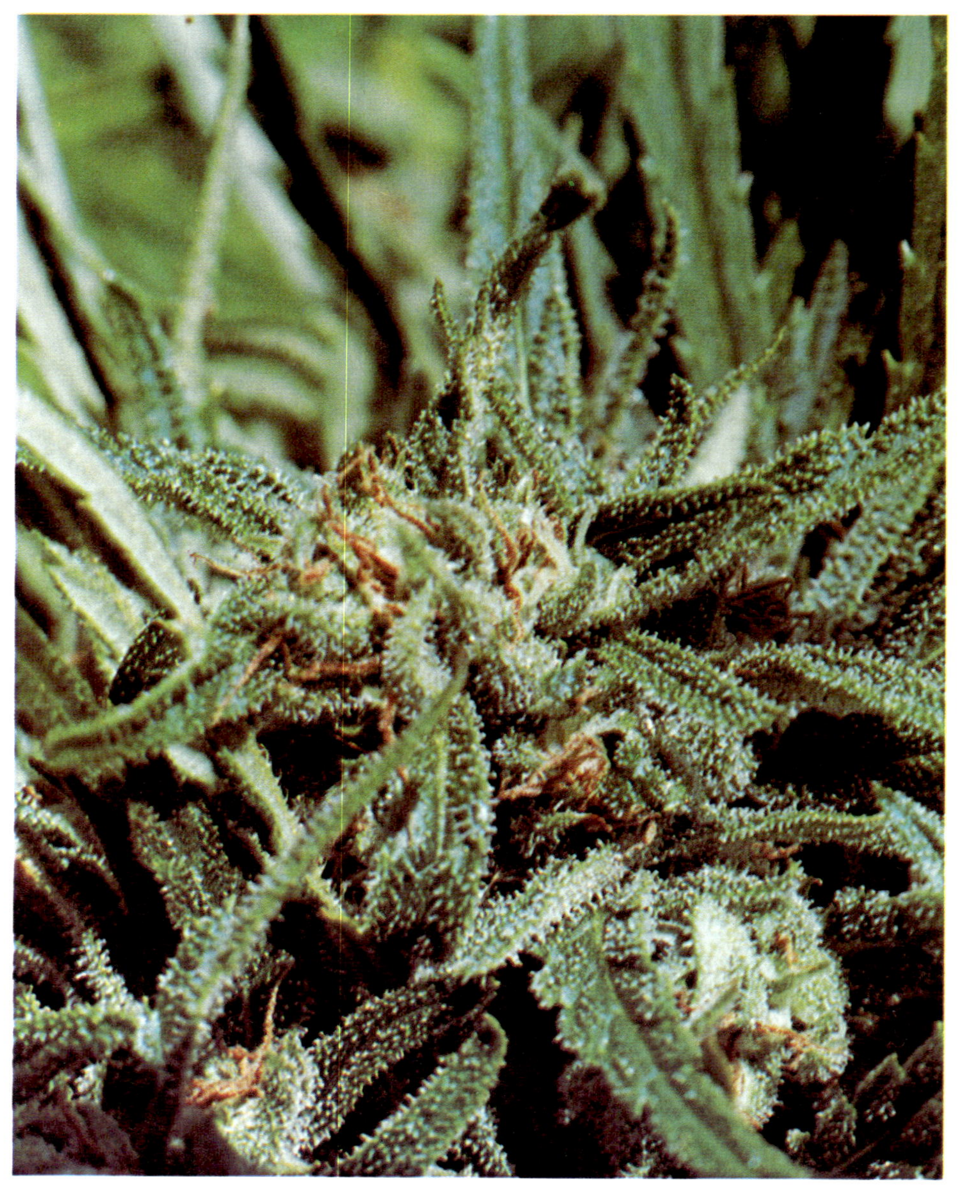

*the pistils brown and fall away—the resin
becomes more coarse on the leaves*

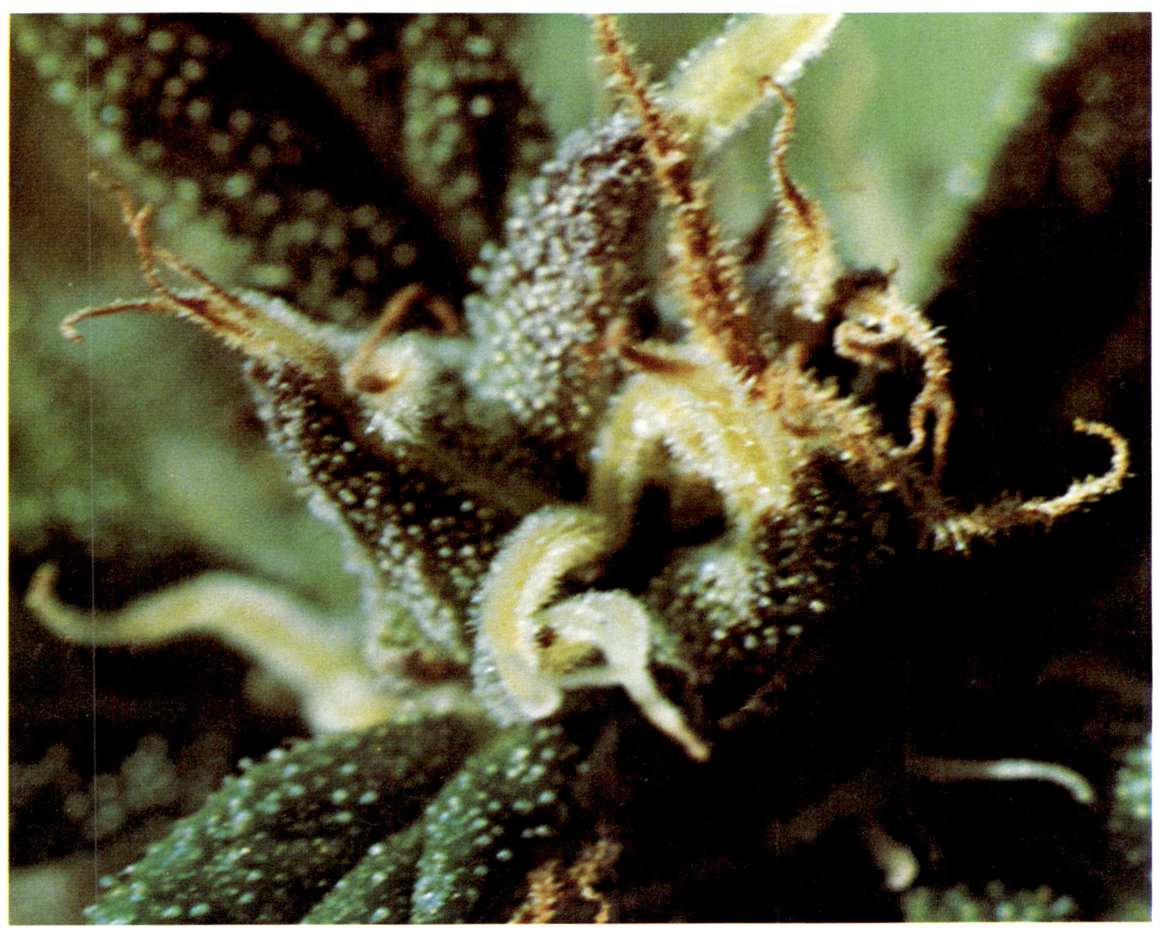

THE FOCUS OF ENERGY becomes diffused as the resin coating spreads outward onto the leaves in the extremities of the clusters. The size and density of the resin particles increases and the globules begin to stand out. This continues until long after the pistils have disappeared and the transformation has become complete—from delicate white blossoms to an anemone-like mass of sticky leaf.

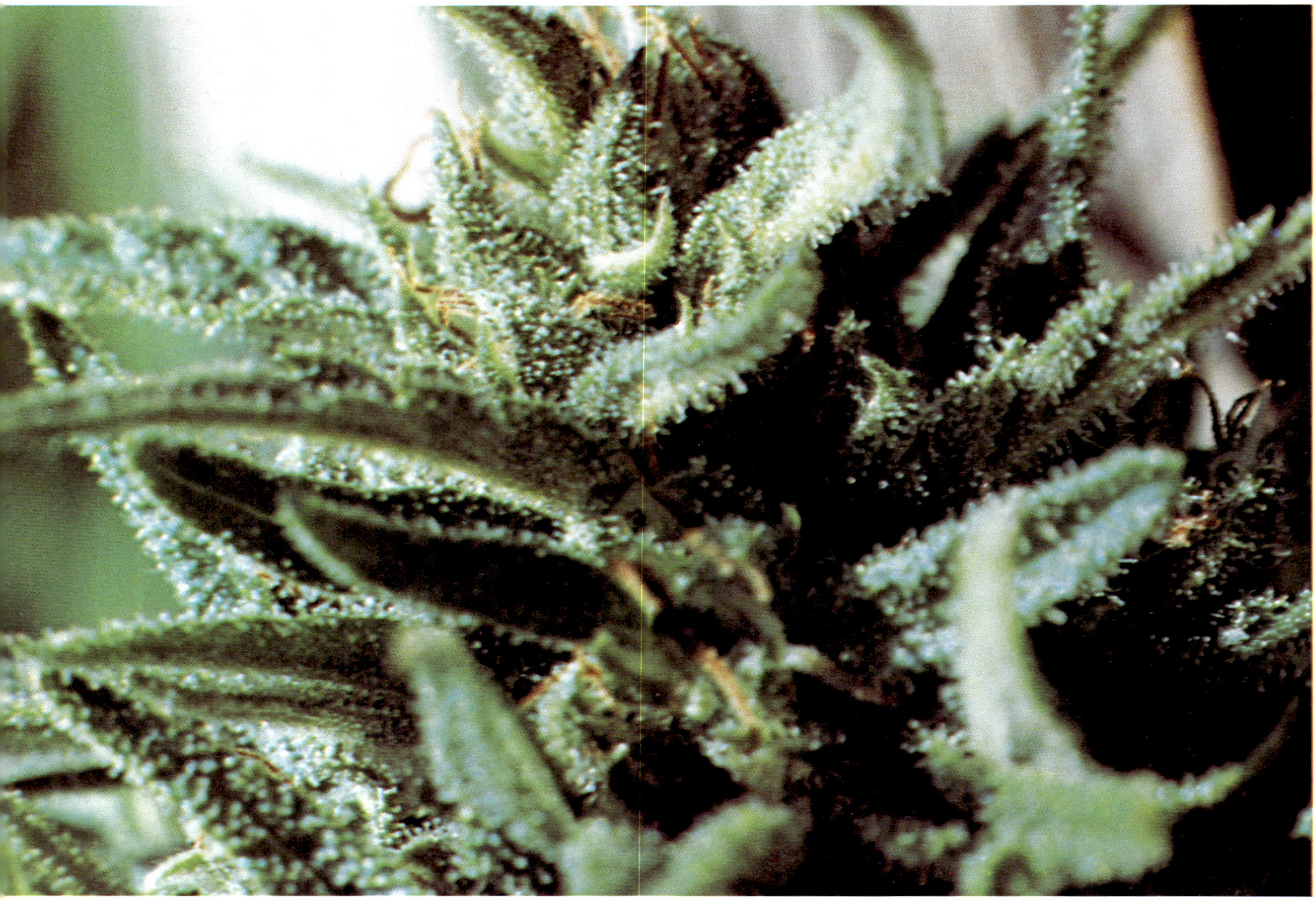

A close-up of the opposite page—here the pistils are almost gone and the colas are incredibly swollen. Compare to the same plant a few weeks earlier at harvest (below).

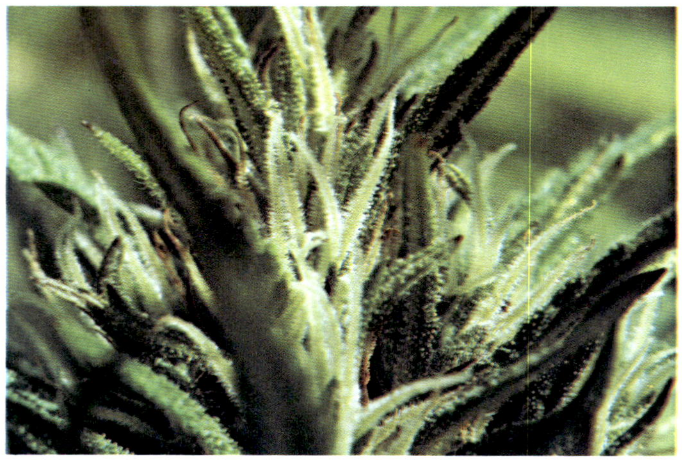

this chrome plating is beautiful but the
sweetness of the sinsemilla is gone

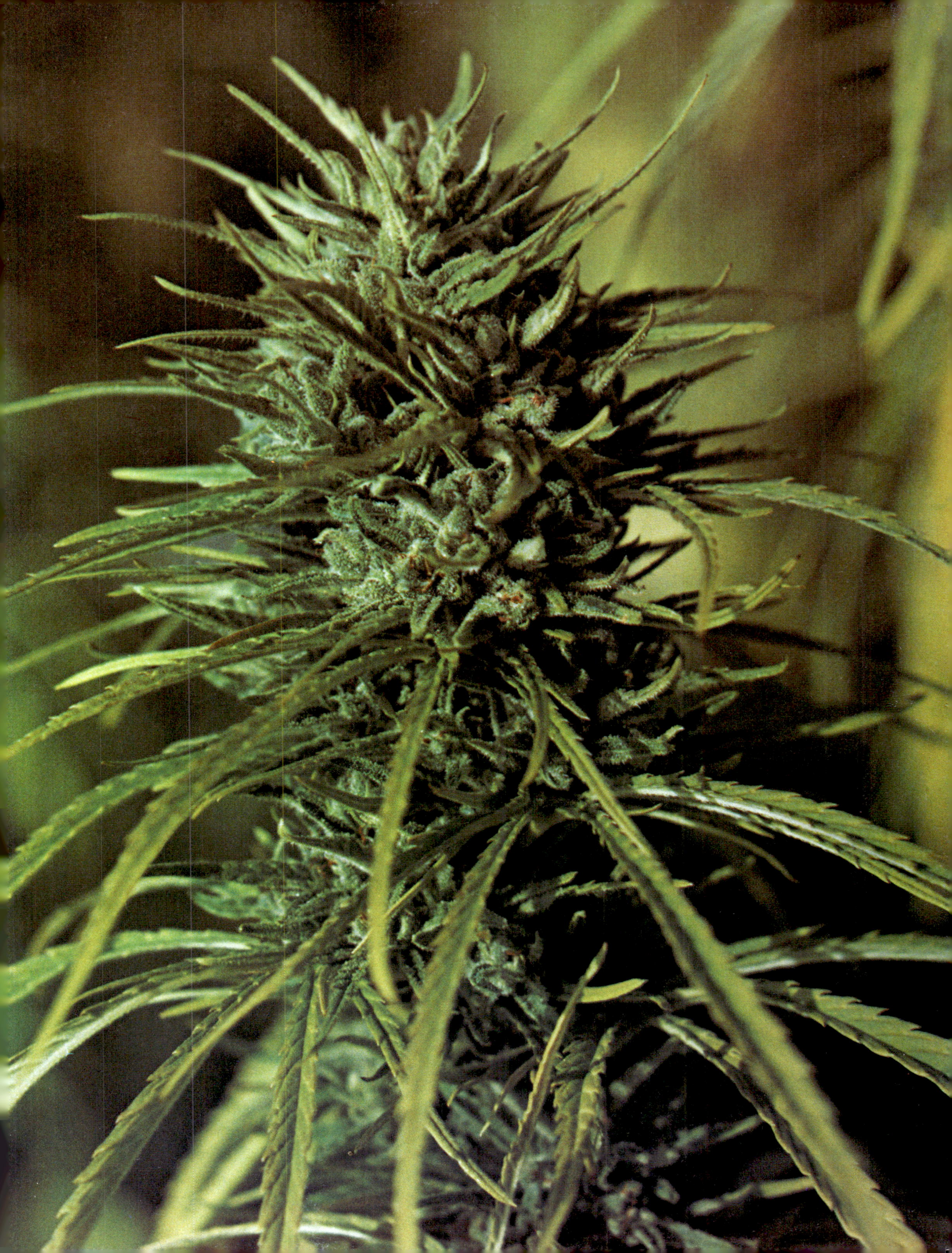

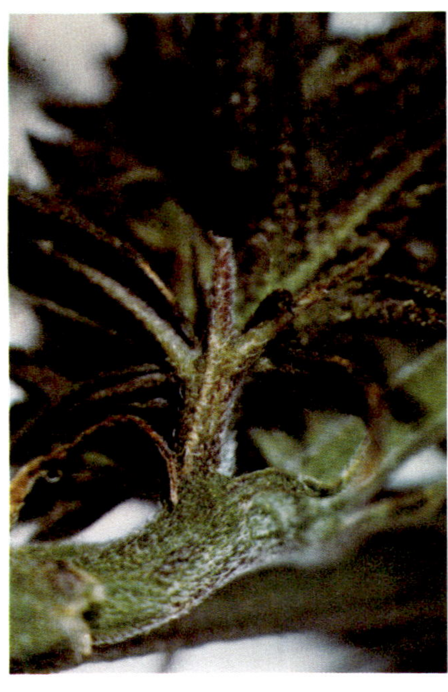

*the underside of some purple
leaves on a green stalk*

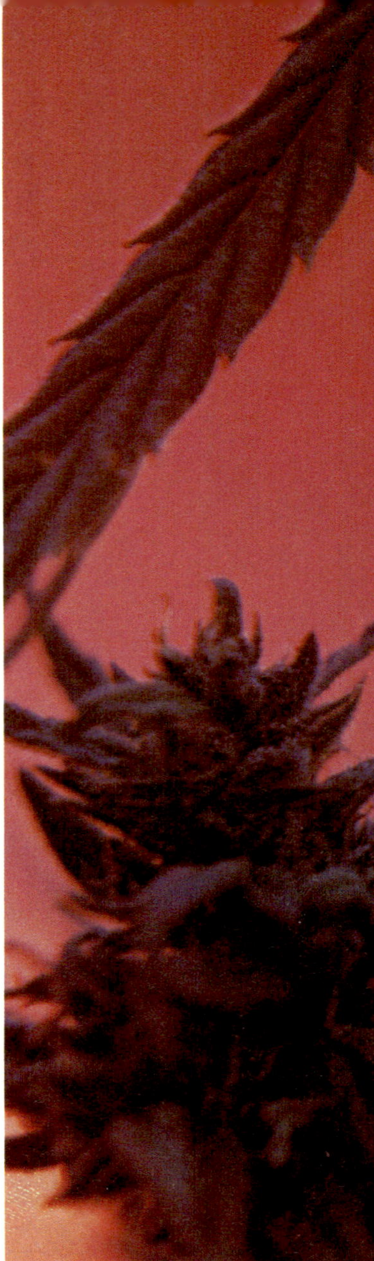

purple stalks with green leaves

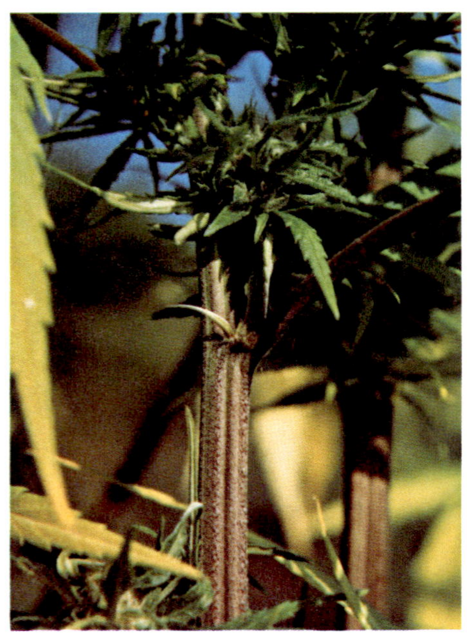

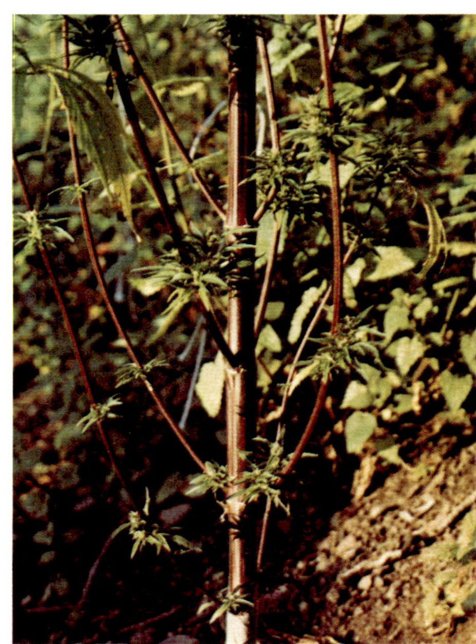

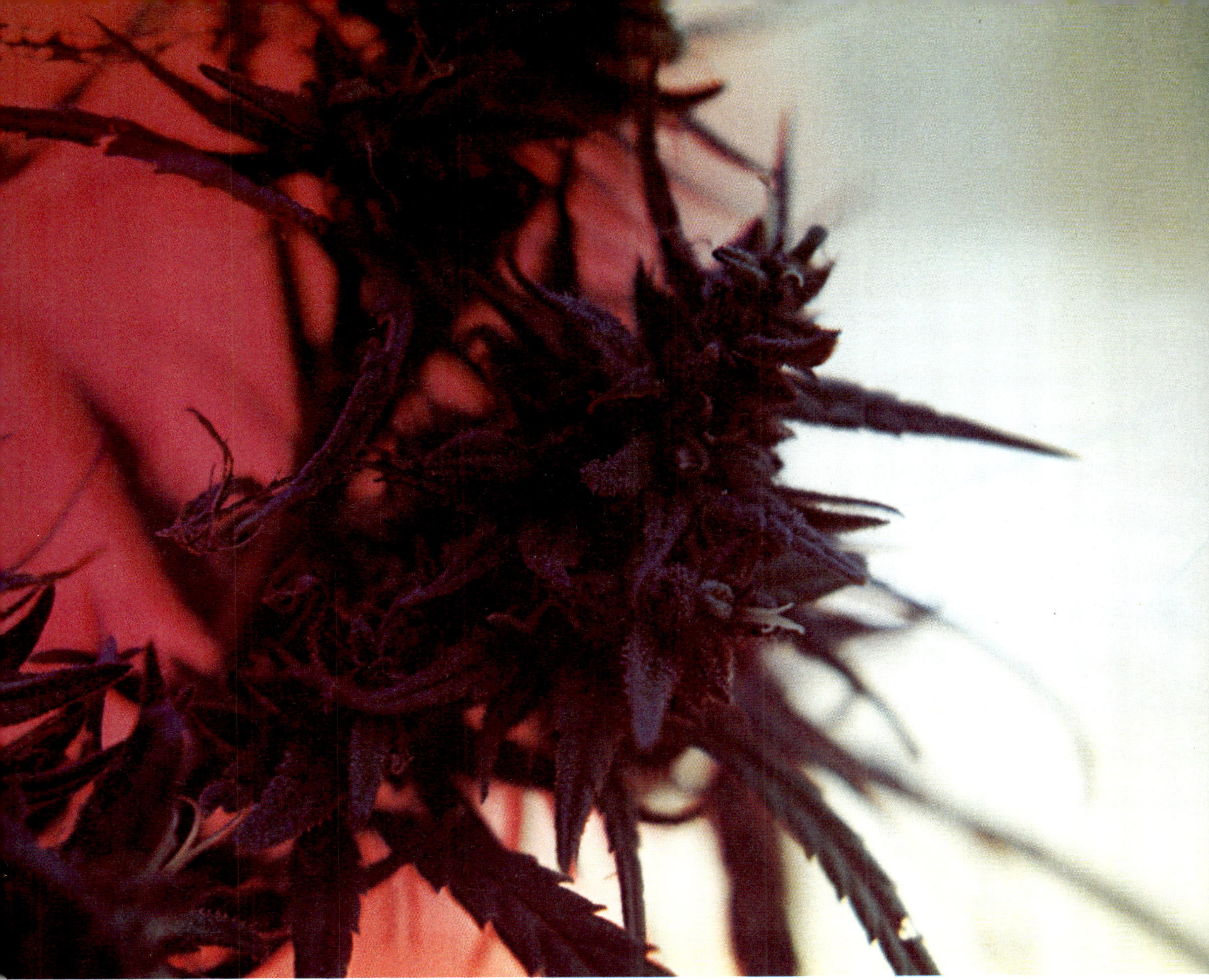

some deep purple flowers long after bloom — a few scattered pistils are still visible

THERE SOMETIMES OCCUR truly purple strains, which as adolescents show coloration in the leaves, on the stalk, and/or in the flowers. However, reds and purples develop more commonly after florescence and this simply indicates the waning of life in the plant, like leaves turning in the autumn. Color does not indicate greater potency in the smoke. Coloration relates to strain characteristics as well as soil and weather. Plants maturing late in cool weather tend to have more colors in the clusters.

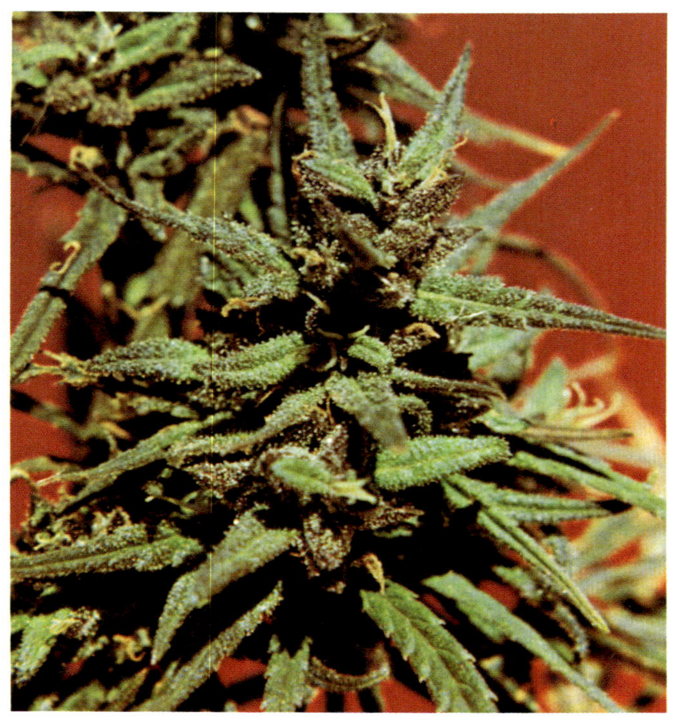

WITH THE PASSING of bloom, the quality of the smoke changes significantly. This is the crux of sinsemilla cultivation and is often misunderstood. Healthy plants from good seed will yield the highest quality marijuana only if harvested at the peak of bloom or soon thereafter. The essential difference between seeded marijuana and sinsemilla is the intense sweetness of the "high." Deterioration of the flowers from extreme age or from heavy pollination yields the same "stoned" effect. If a less stimulating effect is desired, the plants may be left to mature slightly longer after bloom. To some people, the deeper, richer taste is more satisfying, but the sharp edge of the psychedelic may be lost, and it is likely to have more the effect of good seeded marijuana.

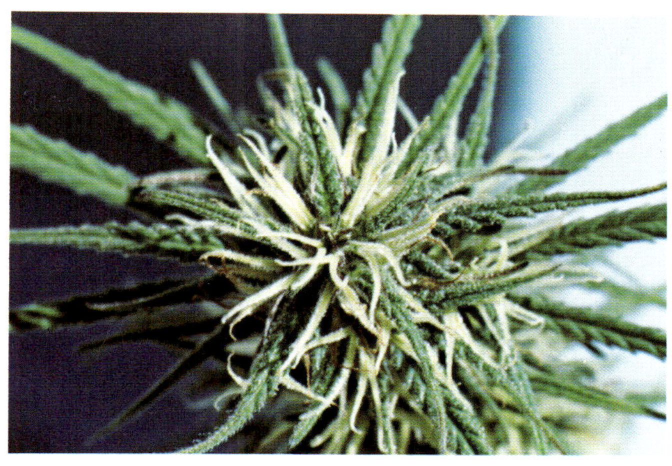

*(opposite) a small late cluster—(below) the tip of the cluster
The empty seed covers have swollen incredibly and turned deep purple,
but the delicacy of the high is gone. Compare to the same plant
at full bloom a few weeks earlier (above).*

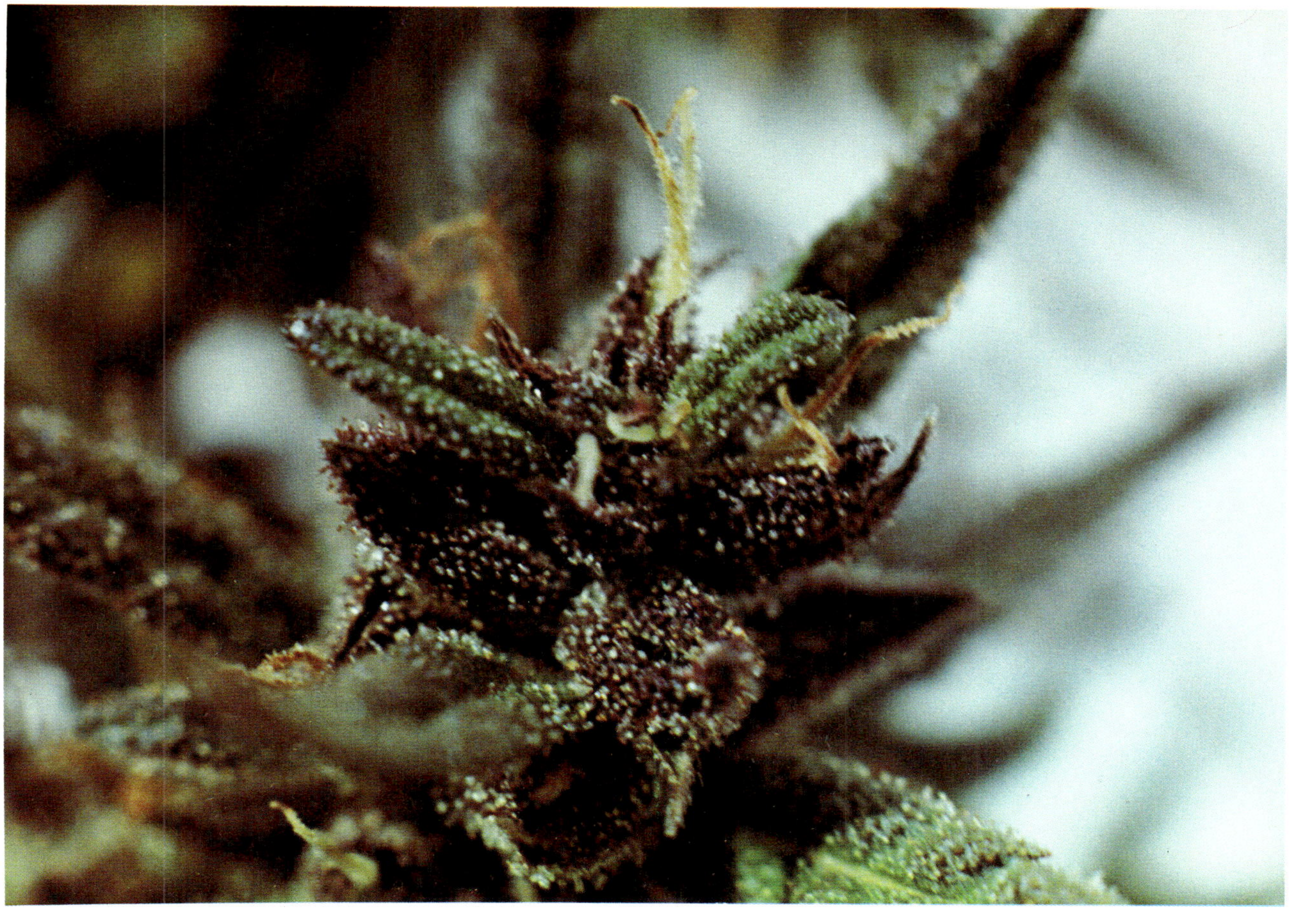

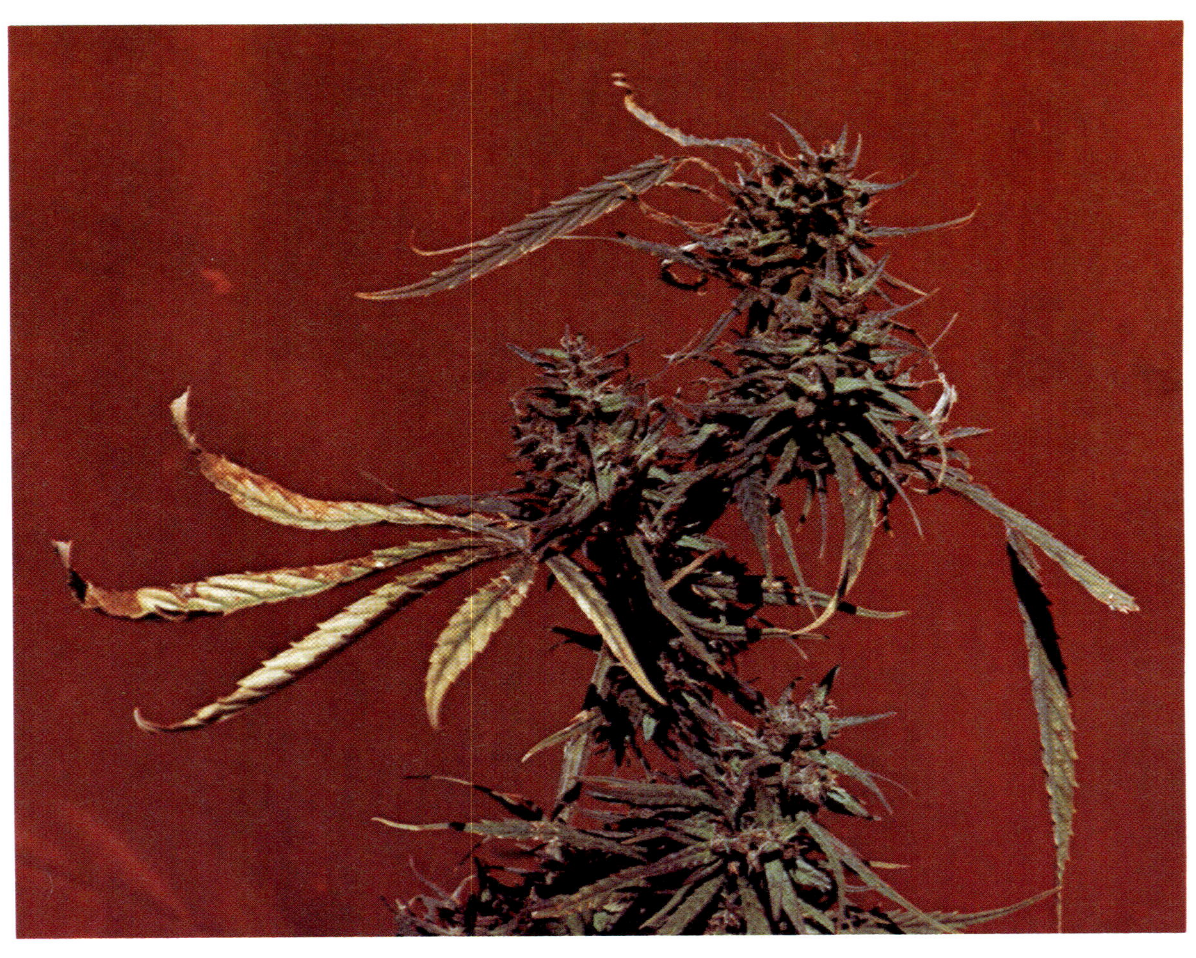

some small clusters left after the large colas have been cut at full bloom

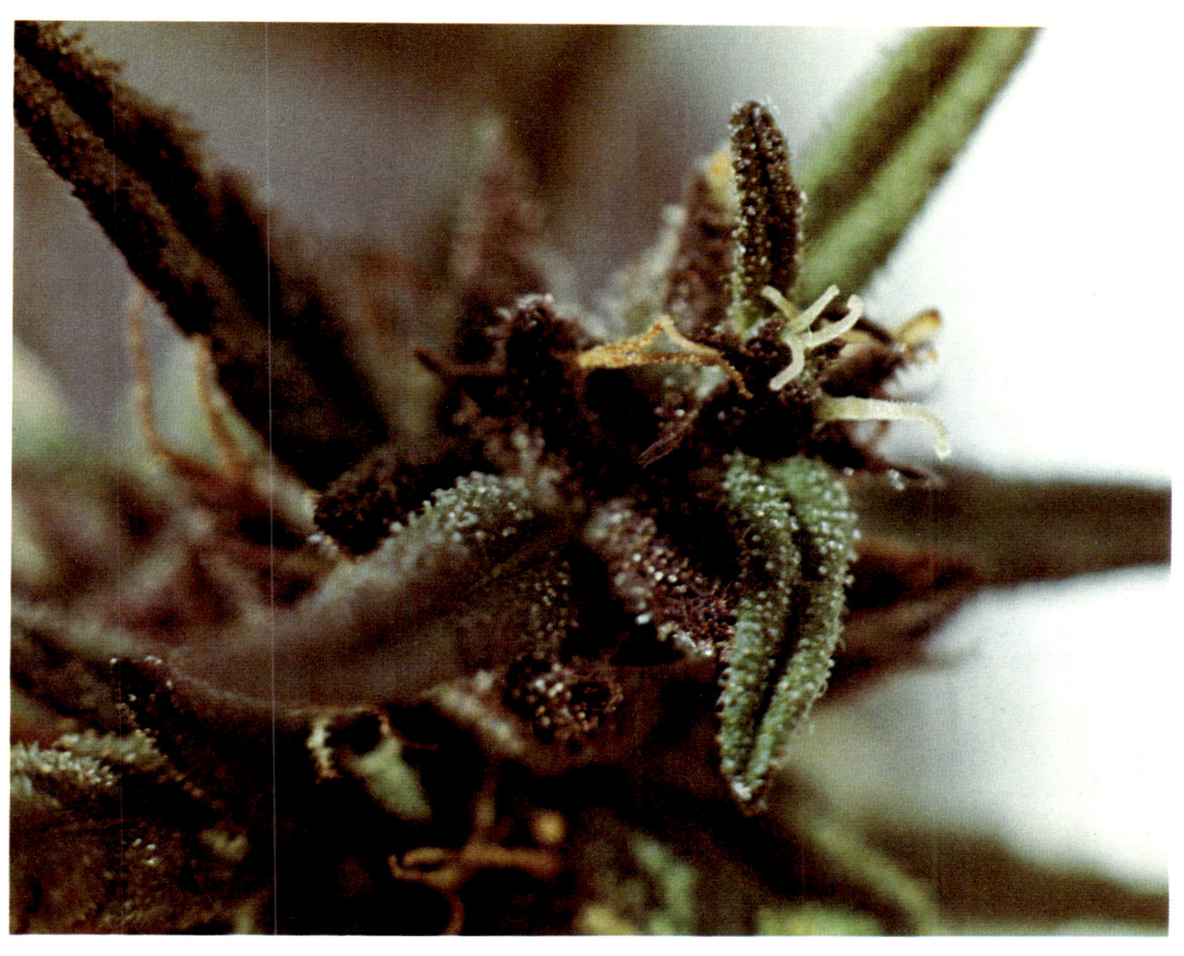

*a close-up of the bottom cluster on the opposite page—a few white pistils
hang on in desperation but most of the blossoms have disappeared long ago*

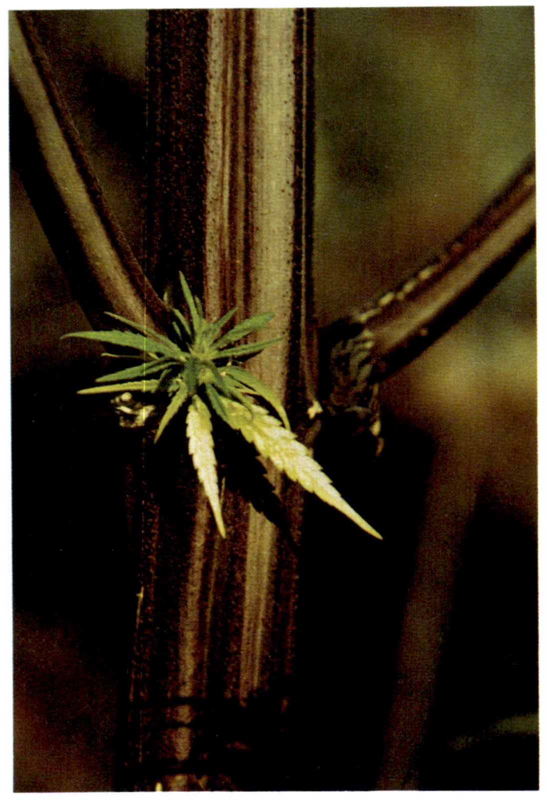

EACH PLANT is different in its flowering pattern, resin build-up and coloration. There is no fixed point for determining the point at which the flowers have reached their peak. Many plants express the classic sinsemilla pattern, all the blossoms climaxing at once. Some varieties have a staggered, drawn-out bloom, in which the older pistils begin to recede and brown early while the pistils in the tips are still green. In some strains, deterioration sets in rapidly after the blossoms are out, while in others the bloom is extended and the flowers retain their potency for a number of days. Weather has a large effect on this variation. Weeks of mellow, warm weather are best for ripening, and cold rain can ruin delicate blossoms.

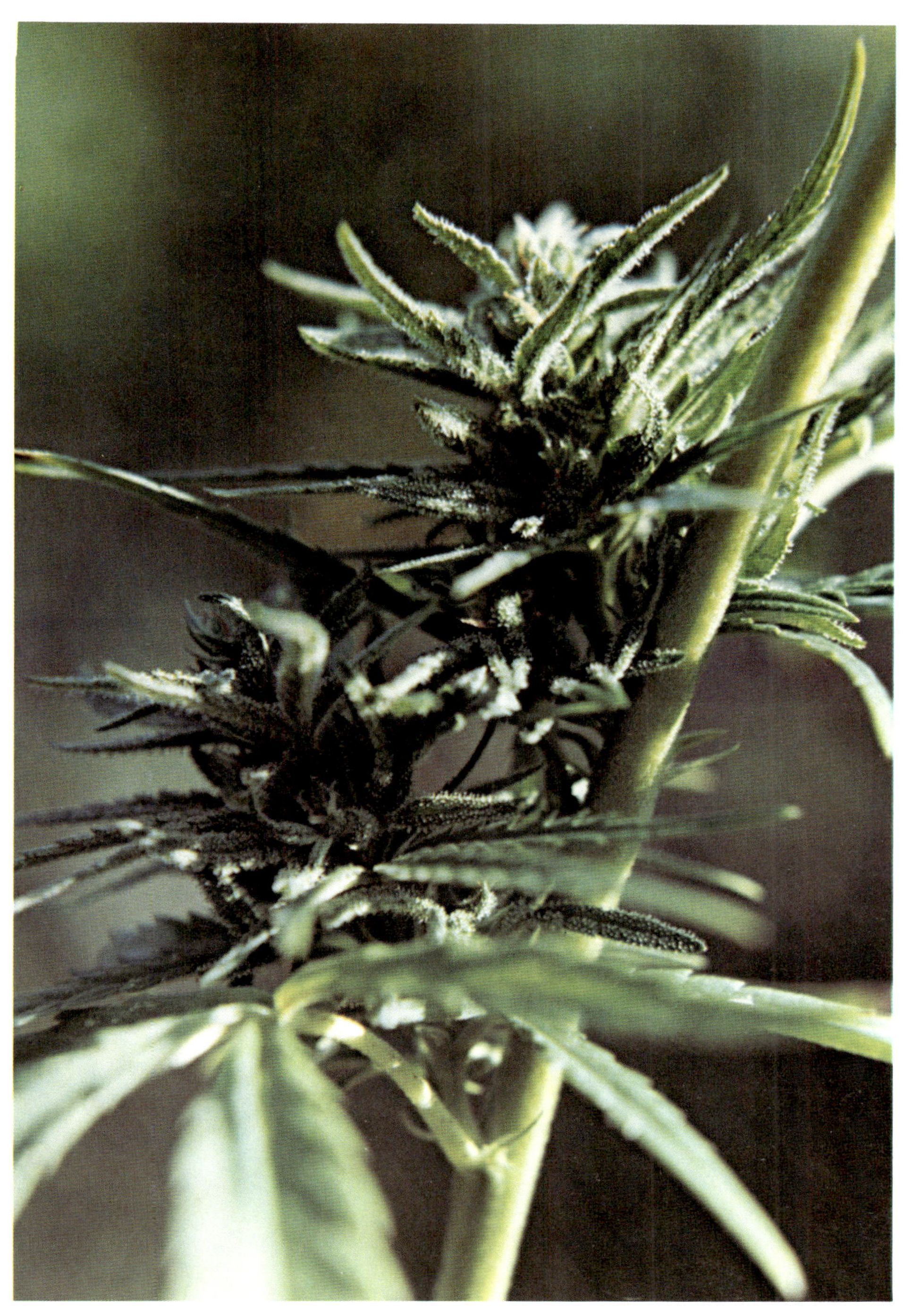

the resin is like snow on the leaves of these late clusters

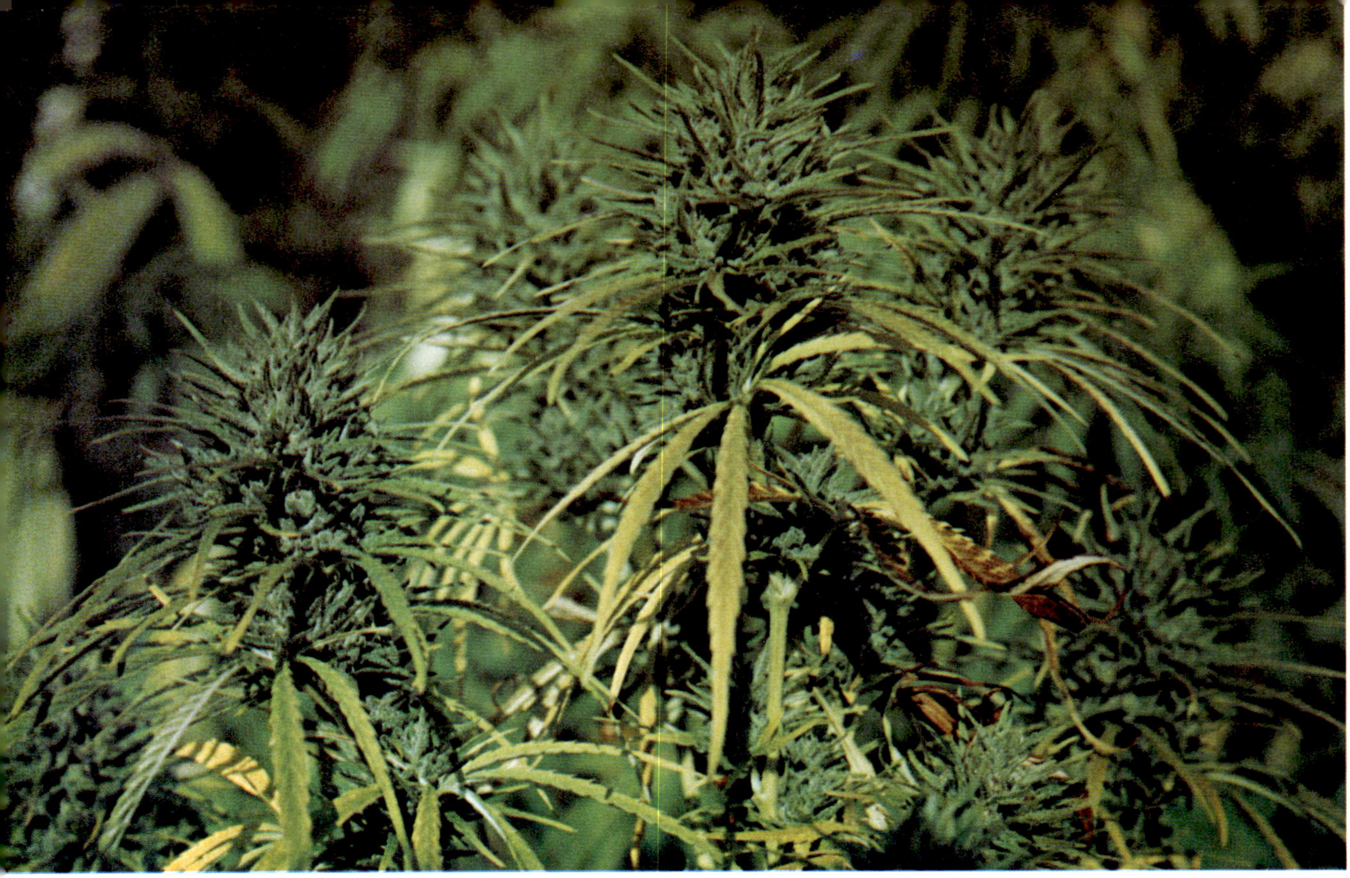

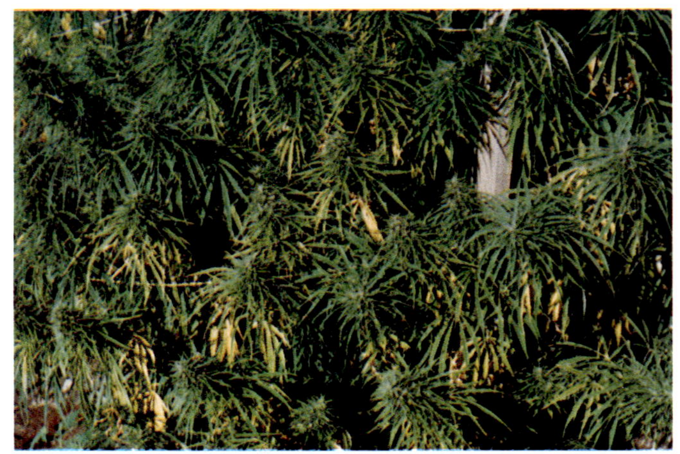

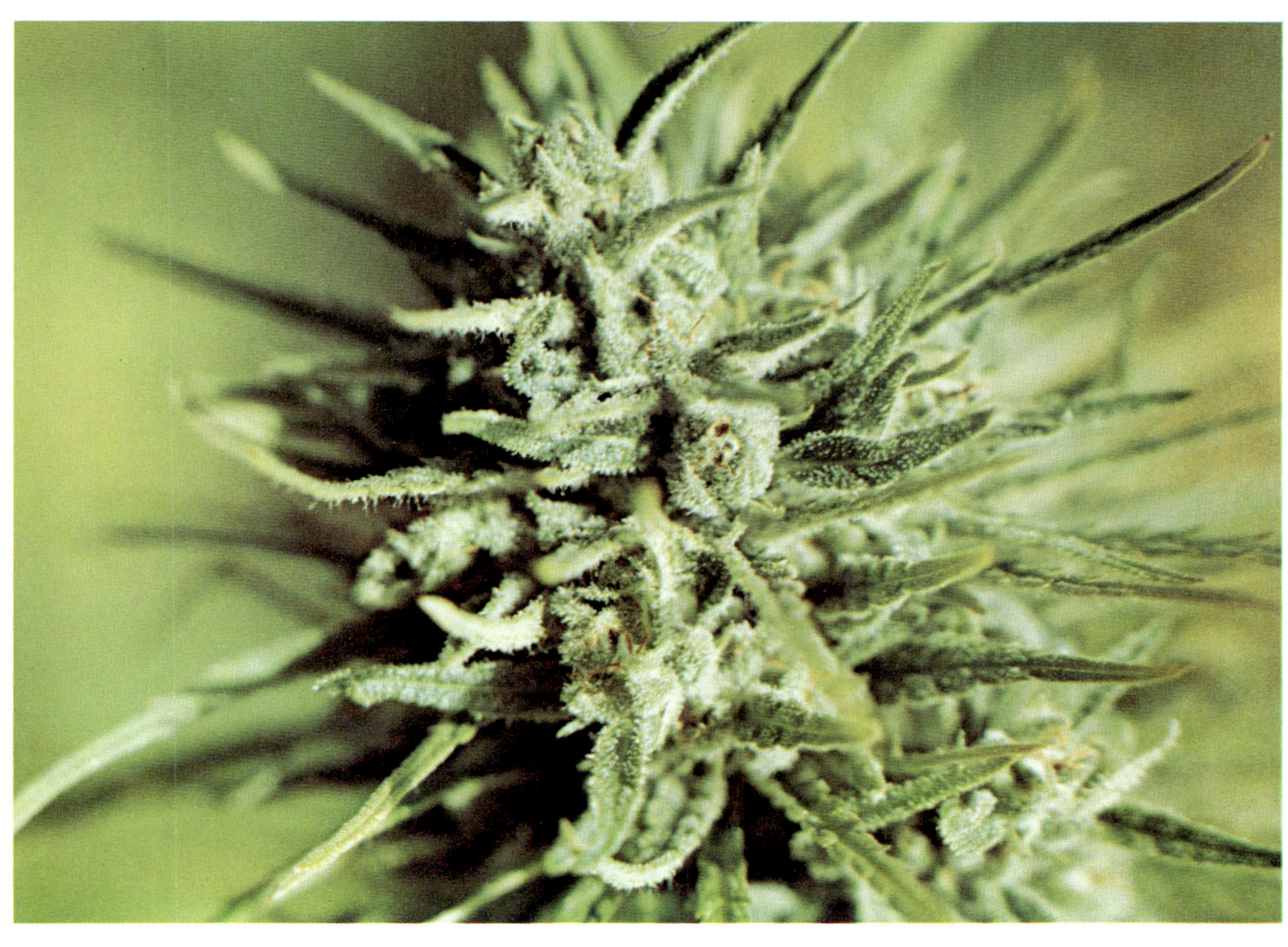

*three views of the same plant—the appearance of huge quantities of resin
after florescence is not an indication of quality smoke*

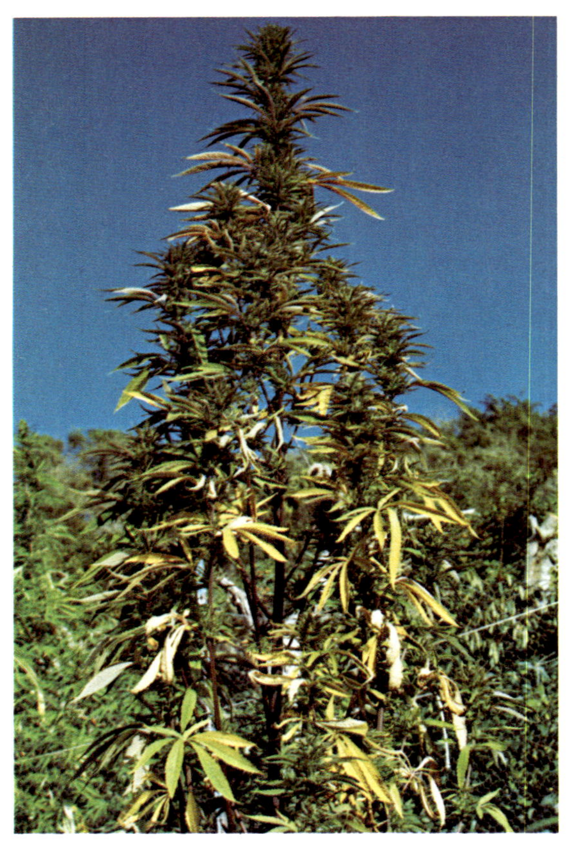

*an old, seedless woman with purple
stalks and yellowing leaves*

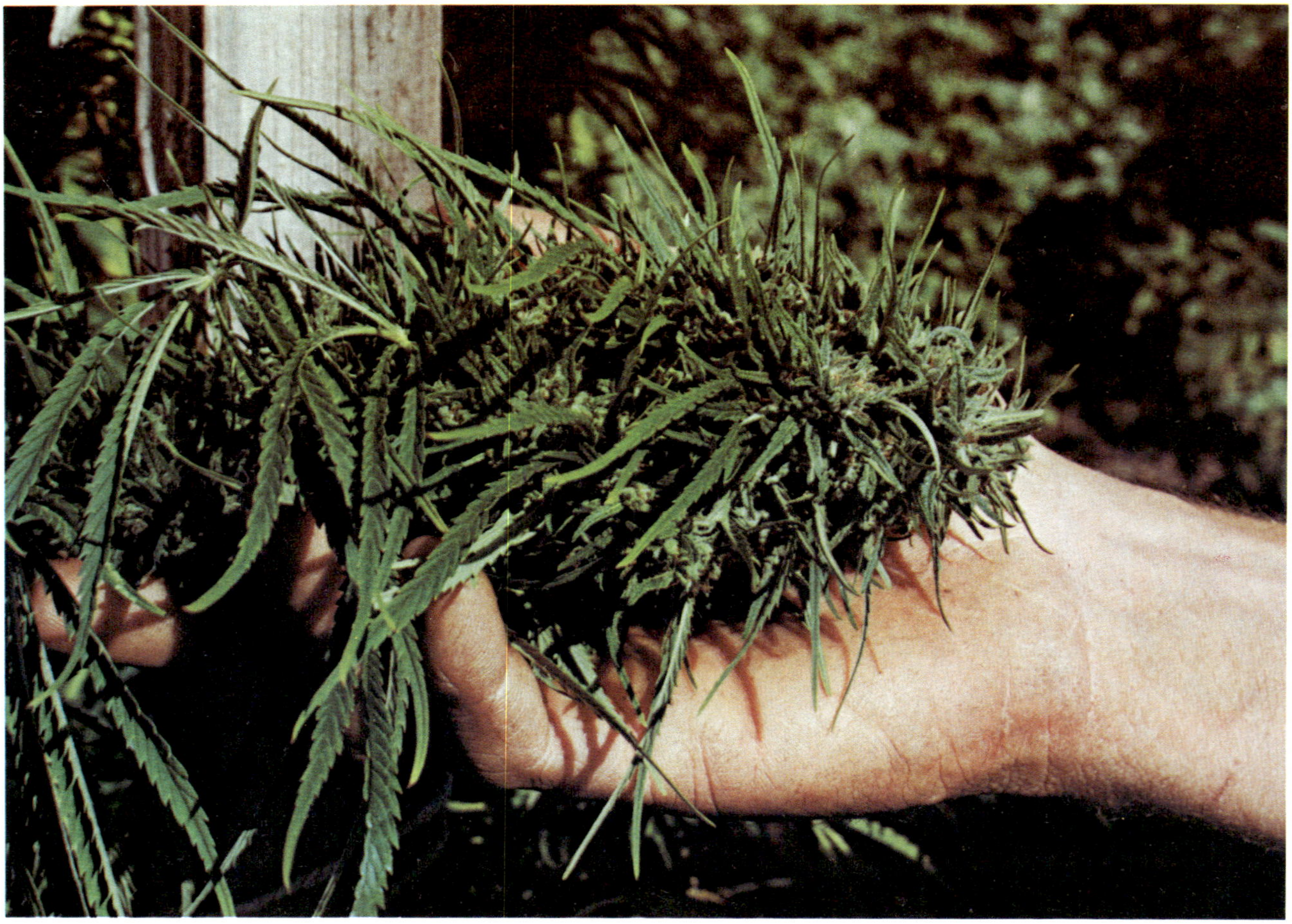

*aged clusters weigh far more than pure flower tops—the weight is in the
thick leaf and heavy resin*

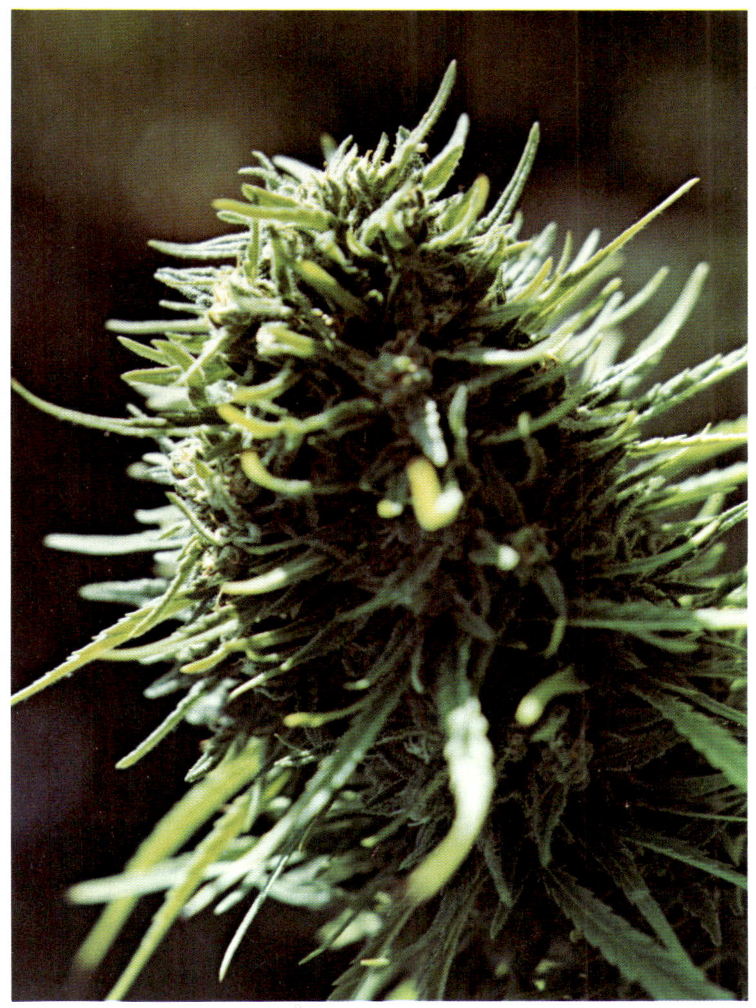

a thick, leafy cola in silhouette

IF THE FLOWERS are to be harvested properly, the rhythm of each plant must be carefully observed during florescence. The scent of the blossoms is the best indication of maturity. The aroma is the quintessence of the herb. Ripe blossoms have an electric sweetness and an ethereal penetrating quality. After the peak of bloom, the aroma becomes more earthy and begins to acquire more body. It gradually loses its lightness and takes on a heavier aspect. The plant is slowly going down, returning to the earth. It no longer aspires upward.

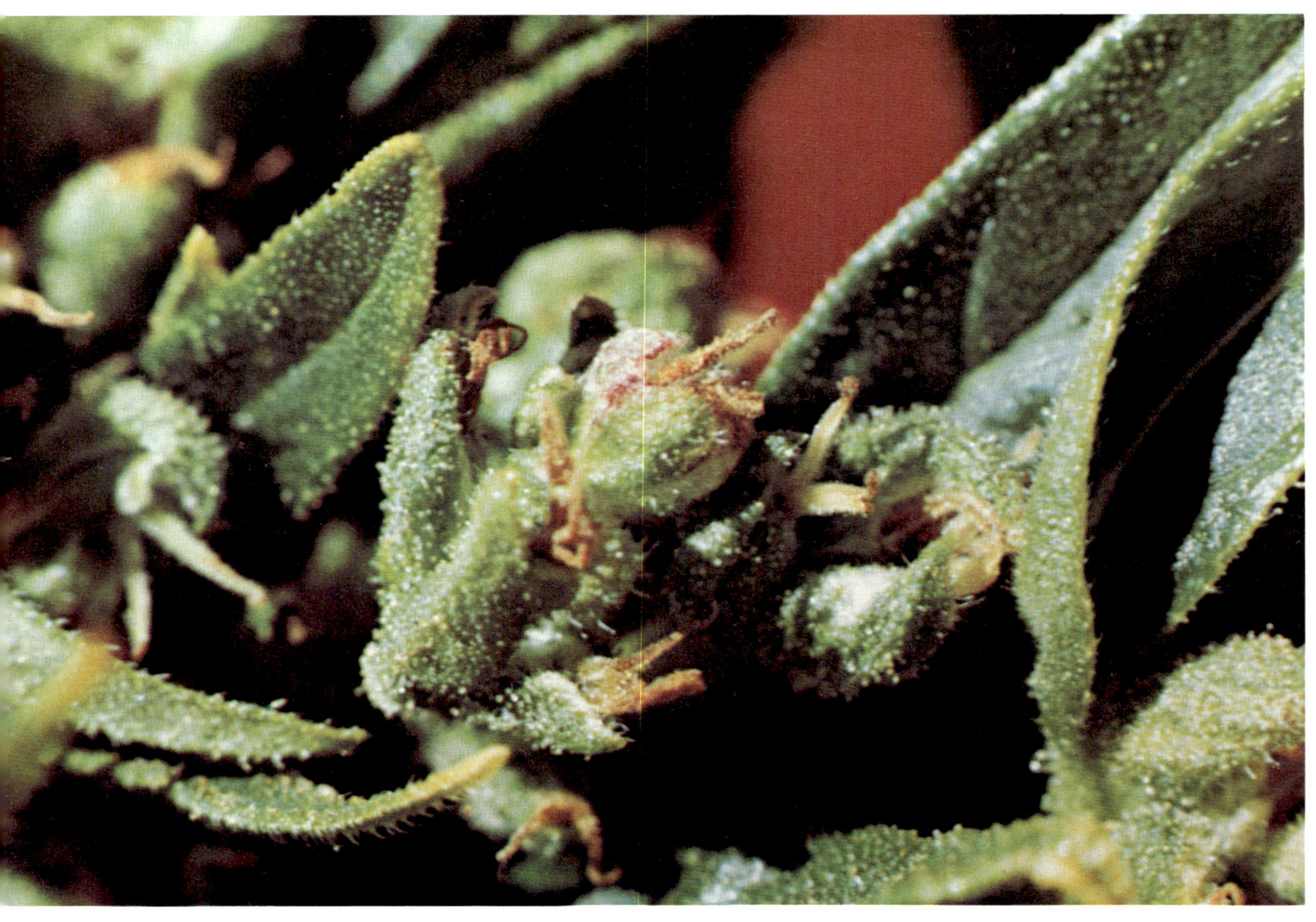

Deterioration is almost complete, but this persistent old plant will not give up hope of pollination. A few pistils remain till the last. Also note the thickness of the leaves and pink in the empty pod at center. See the same plant a few weeks earlier (pages 58, 59).

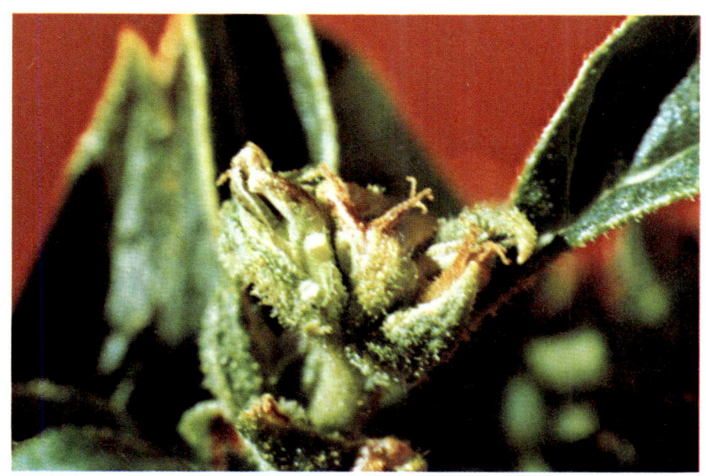

*in the end, the unpollinated flowers
turn back into leaf*

WHEN LEFT UNHARVESTED, the seedless clusters revert into leaf-like structures. The plant finally gives up hope of reproduction and turns in upon itself and dies. Occasionally, in a mild climate, if enough leaf is left uncut, a late maturing plant will retain a bit of green through the winter and may come alive in the spring. But the cannabis is by nature an annual and a two year plant is an exception. It will rarely be as vigorous as a plant started from seed in the spring.

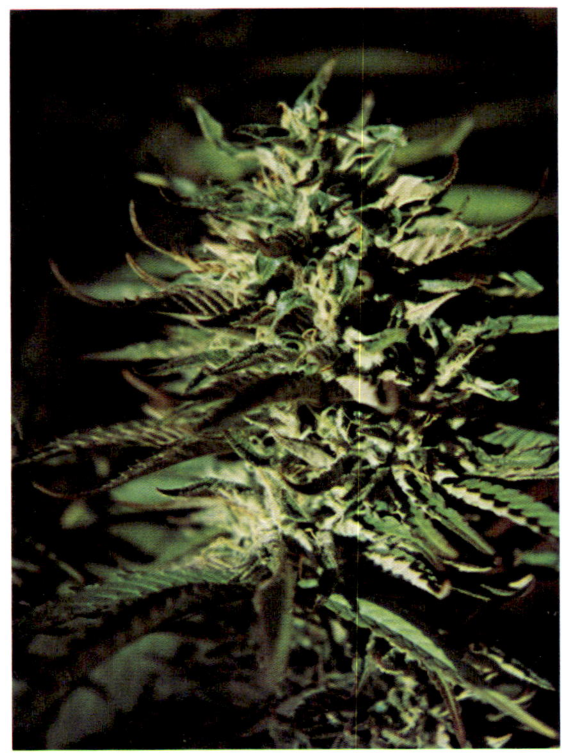

some leafy rogue varieties

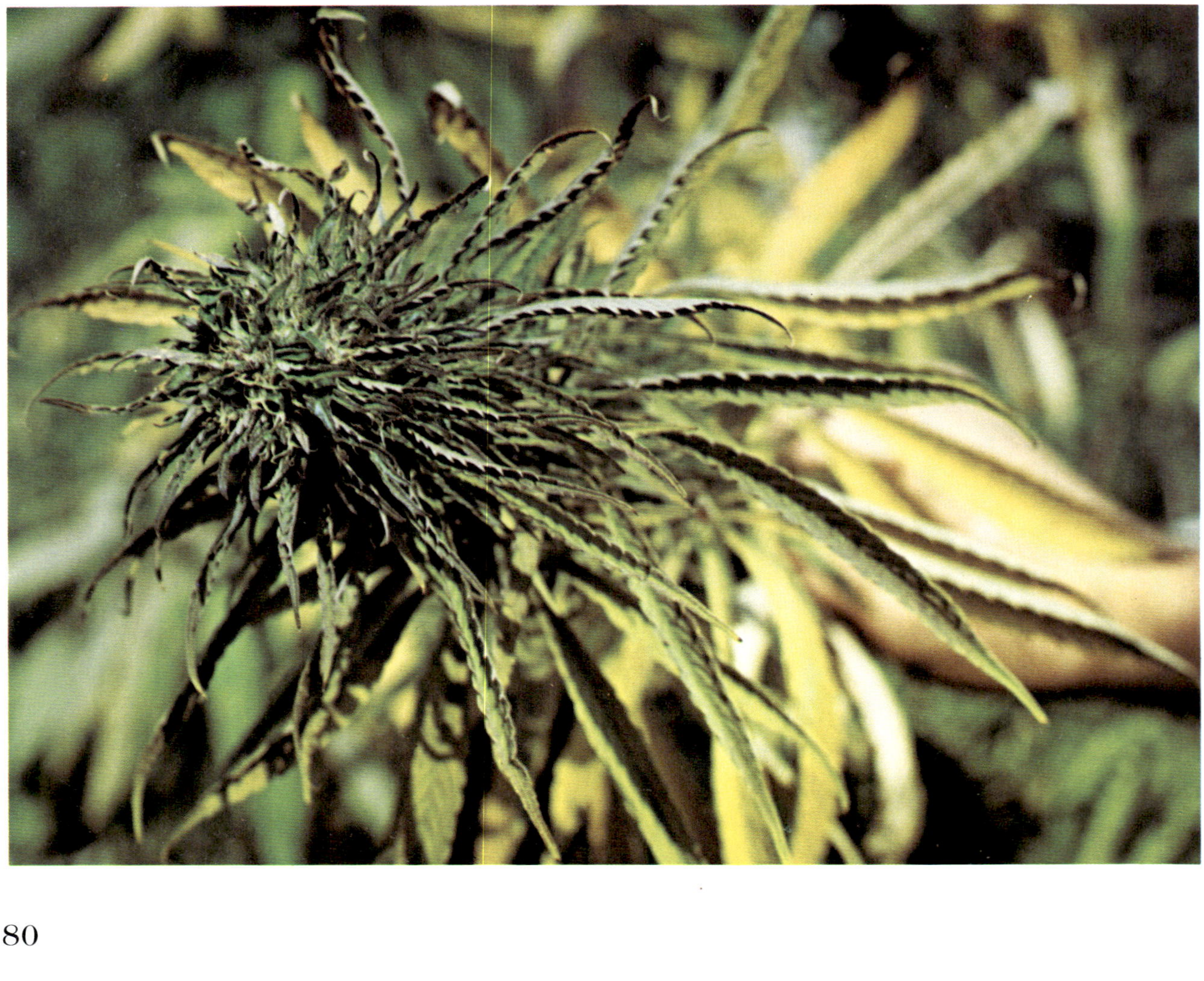

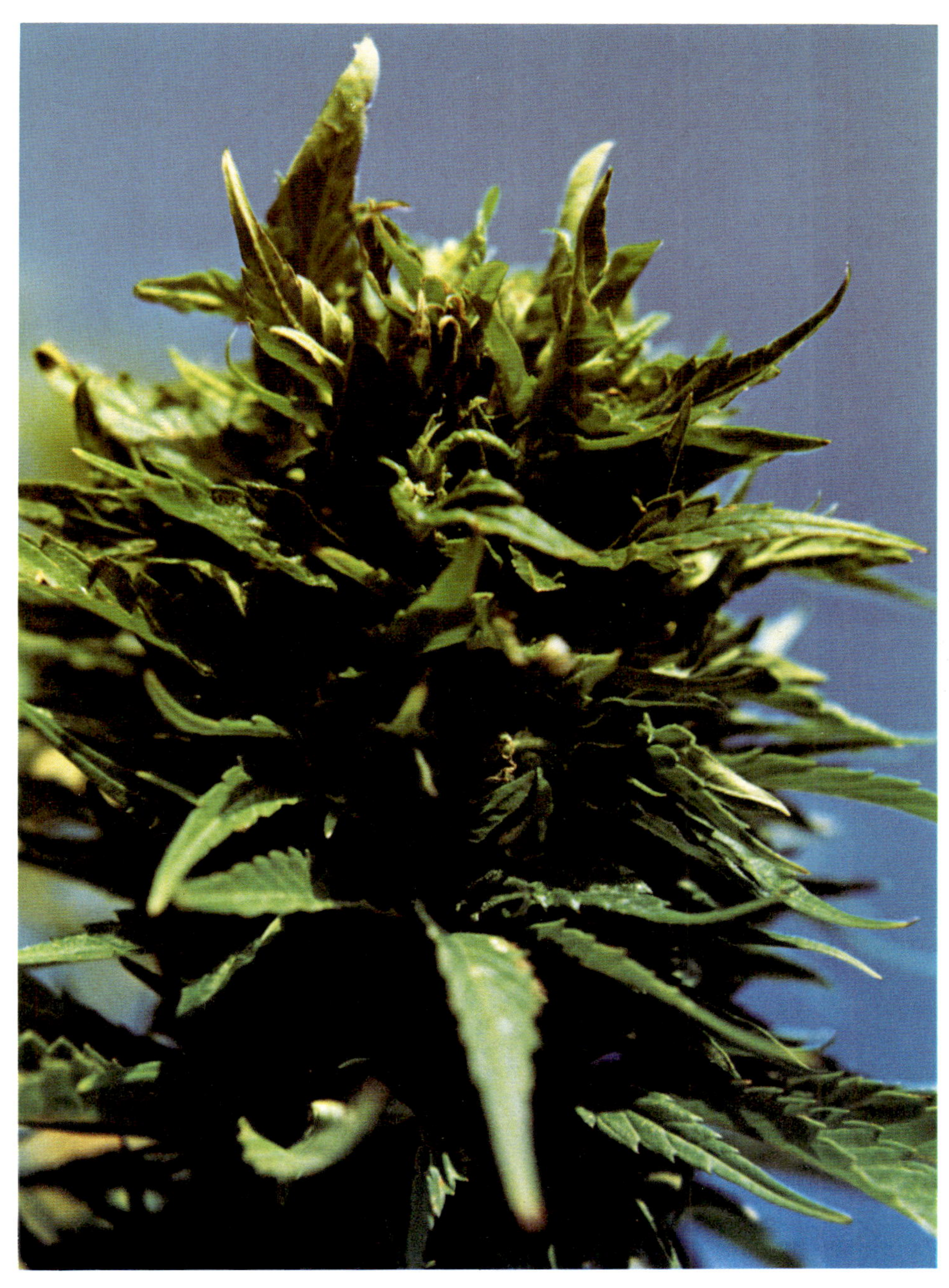

SINCE THE RIGHT of pollination is denied the plant, some degree of hand pollination may be done to make seed for the next year. Specific plants or branches may be carefully dusted with a small branch of a distant or severely pruned male. Care must be taken since a single flowering male can ruin many sinsemilla plants.

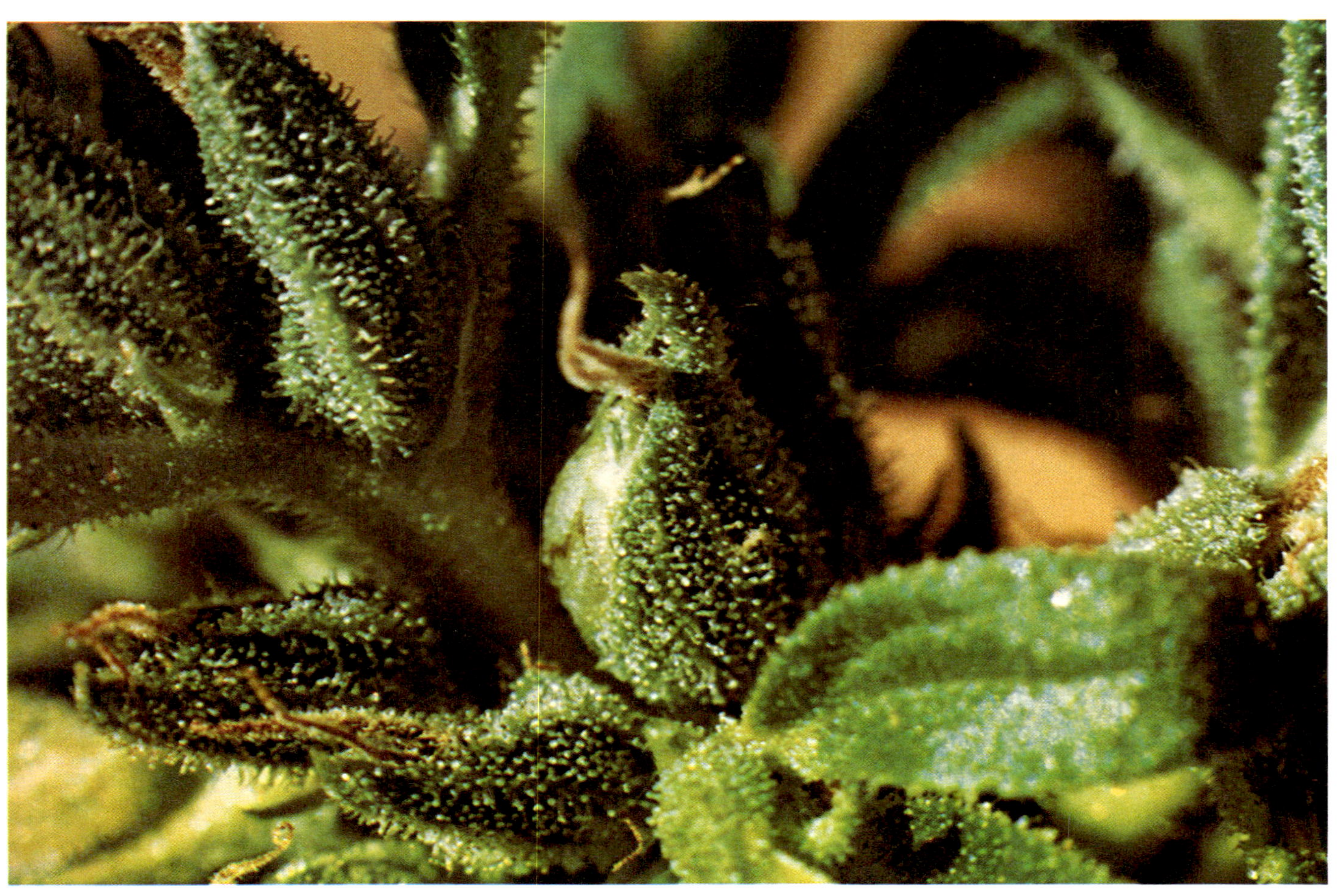

*a lone seed surrounded by aged, unpollinated flowers—for viability
the seed must be allowed to ripen fully*

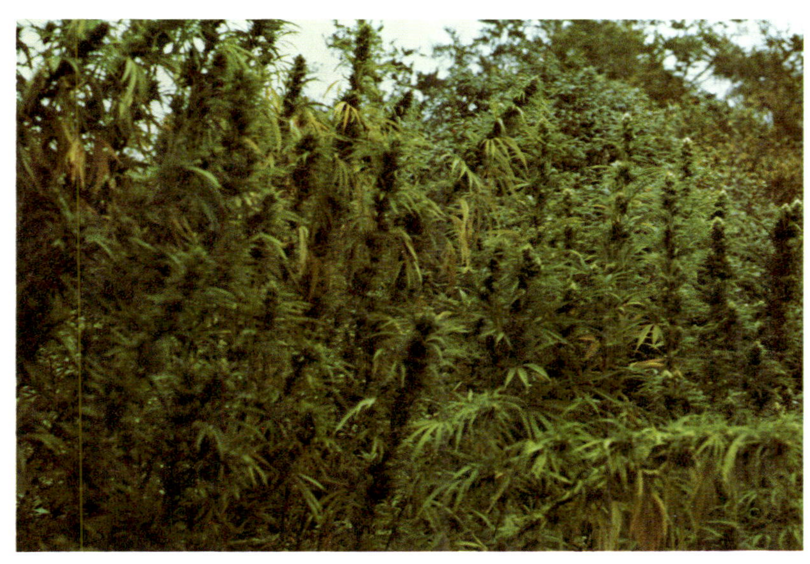

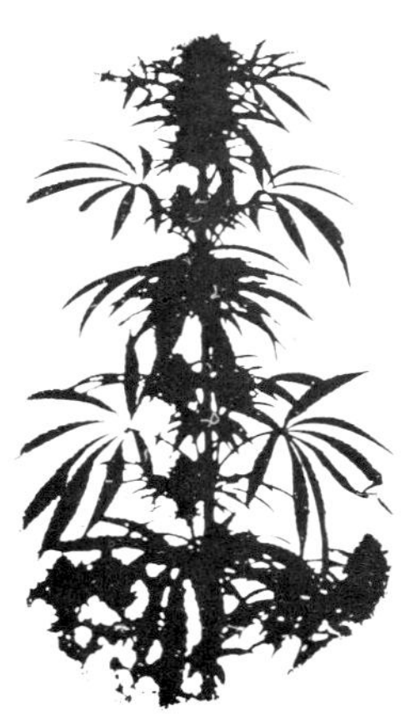

PART FOUR

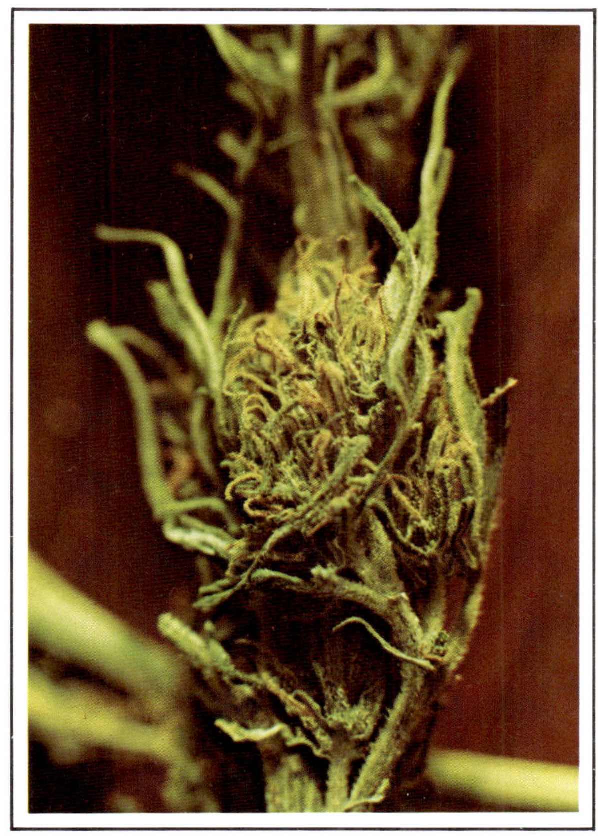

THE SMOKE

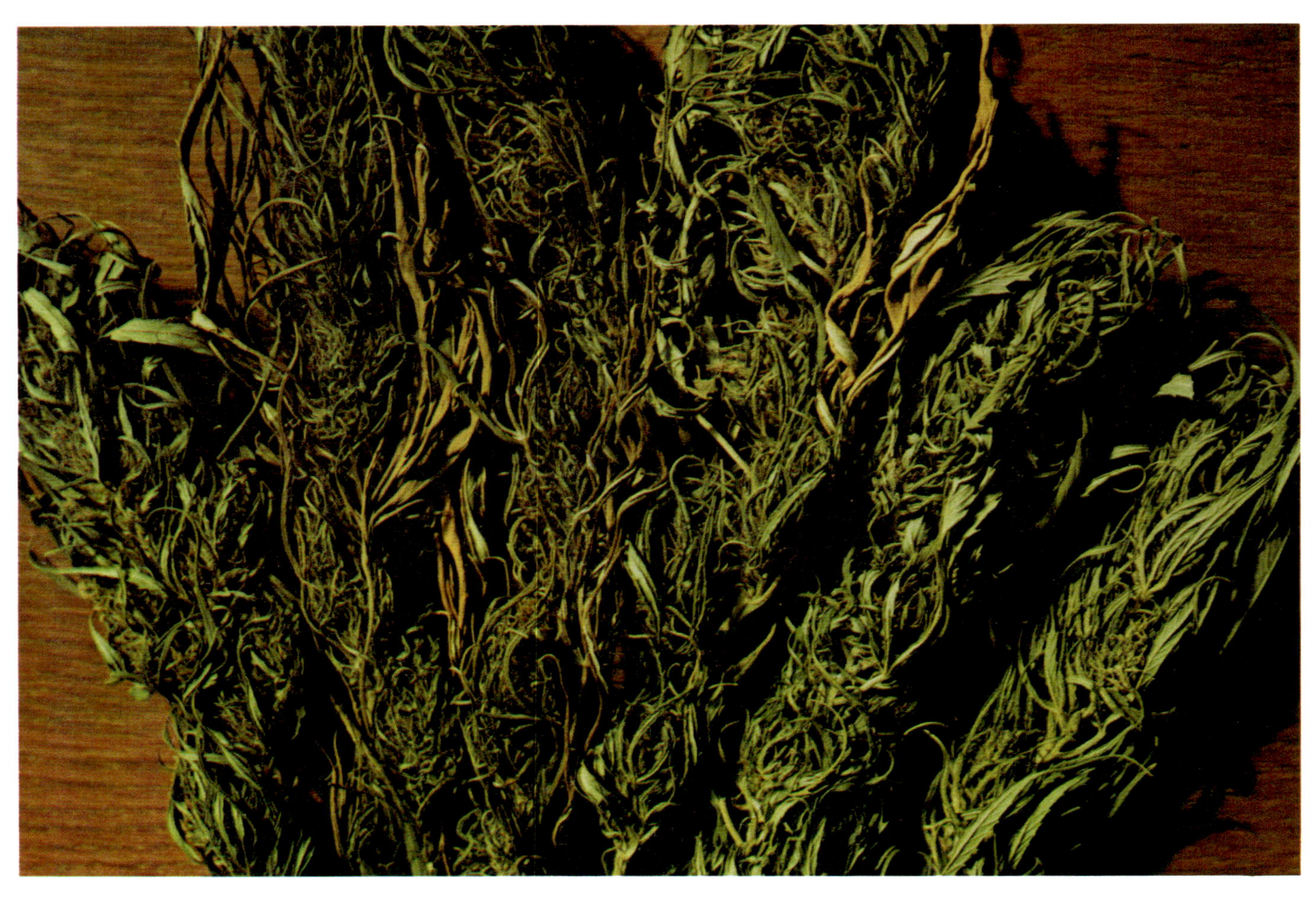

*a selection of dry colas from different plants before the fan leaves are trimmed
It is difficult to see the flowers beneath all their clothing.*

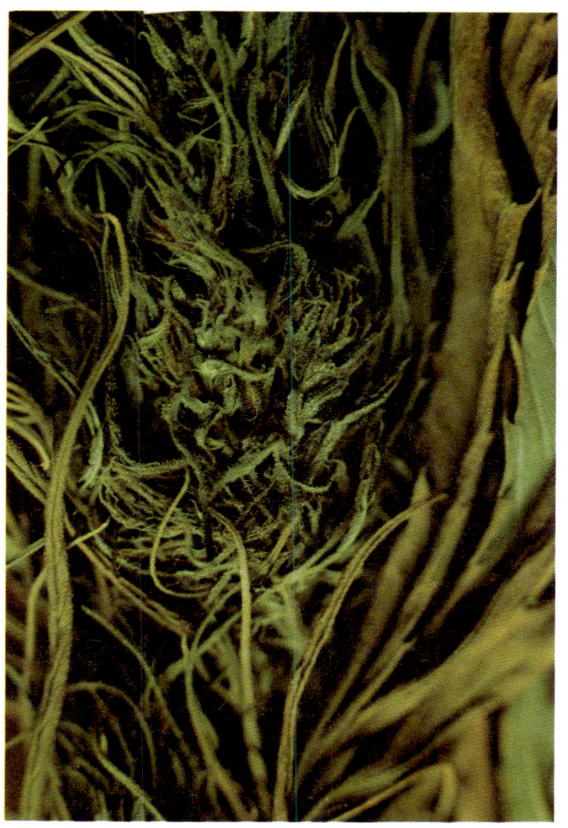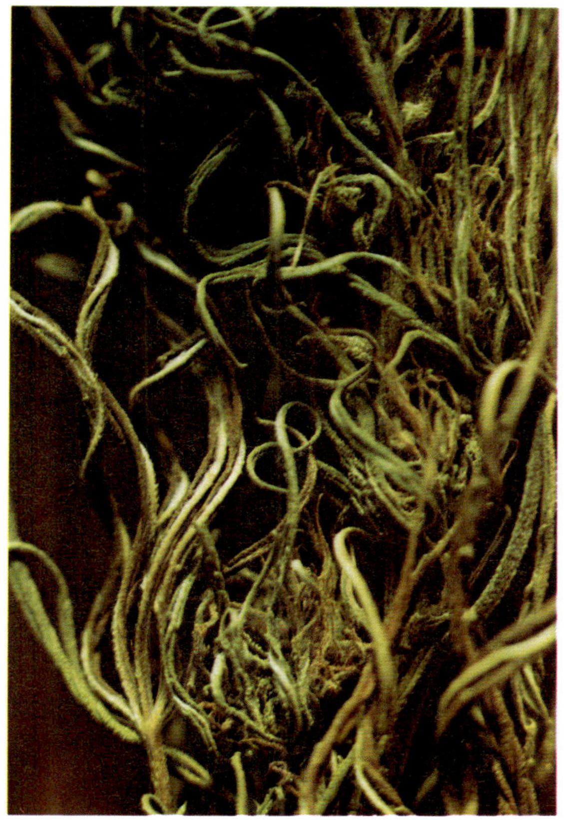

AS SOON AS THE COLAS are taken from the plant, they begin to wilt and lose their brillance. As they are handled, they release their perfumes and a fine resin dust falls to the ground. This is best avoided for the flowers should be preserved in as nearly a life-like state as possible. Any form of multilation may detract from the potency and sweetness of the blossoms.

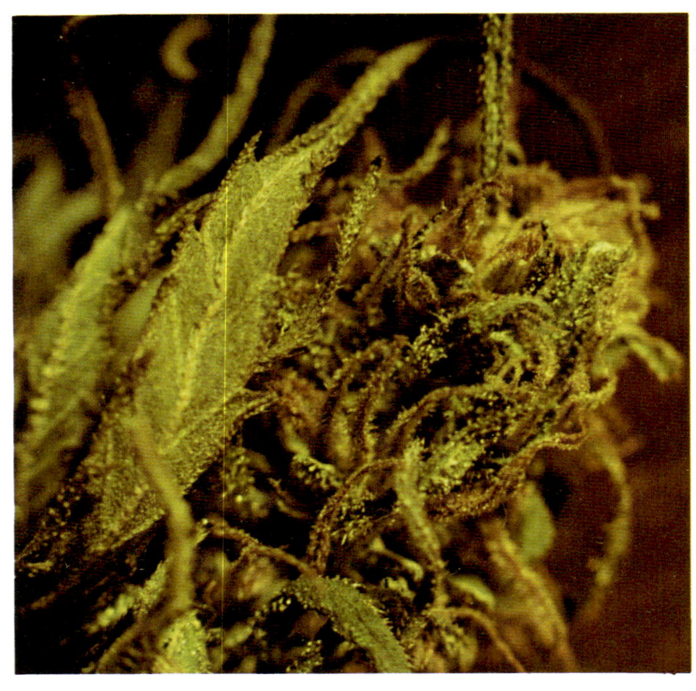

the golden flowers on these two pages
come from colas on page 41

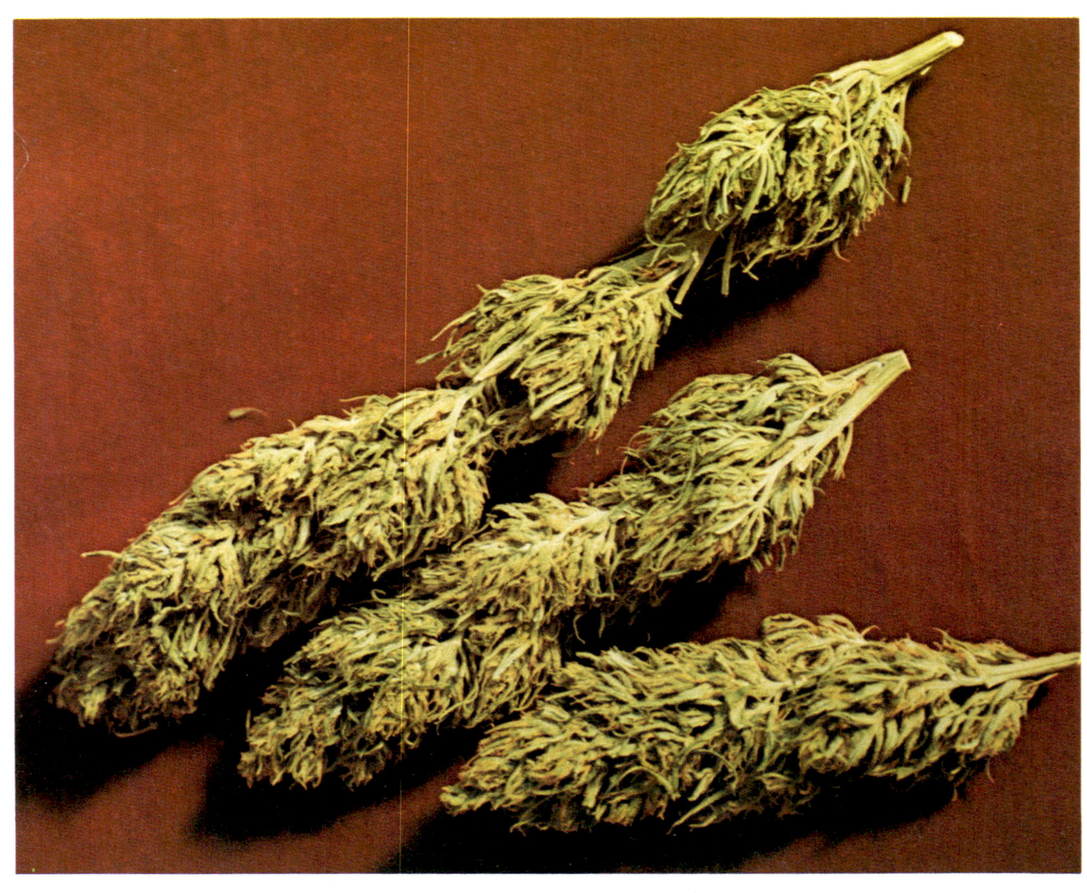

THE MOST CONCENTRATED SMOKE is in the pistils, empty seed covers and minute leaves in the centers of the clusters. Extraneous leaf tends to dilute the clarity of the "high" and carries with it a harshness in the smoke. To attain the pure essence of the flowers, most of this leaf may be deleted from the preparation. In extremely leafy varieties, this may be impossible (see pages 80, 81). The ideal plant has dense clusters of flowers alone (see below).

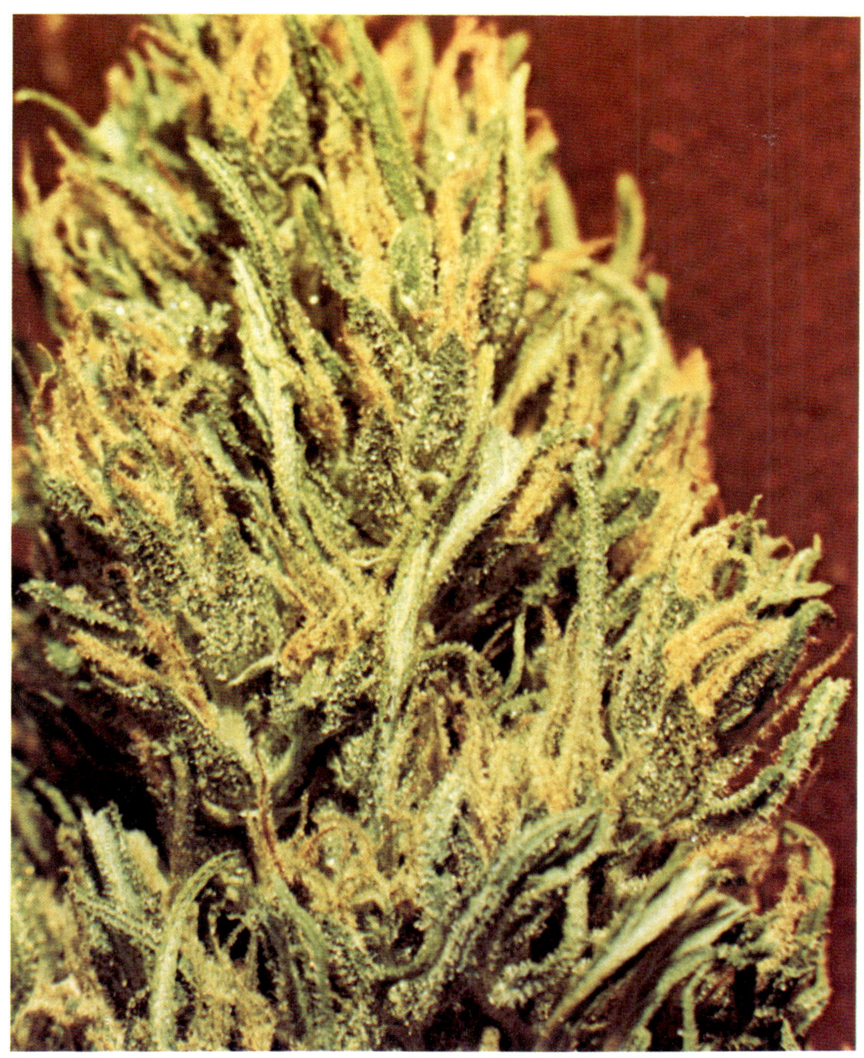

IT SHOULD BE CLEAR that there is no need for gimmickry in the curing process. At this point nothing can be done to improve the quality of poor marijuana, while fine sinsemilla can be ruined by careless methods.

These flowers came from the plants on page 35 and may be seen again on page 55.
The purple colas on page 68 are the small clusters left on the plant after harvest.

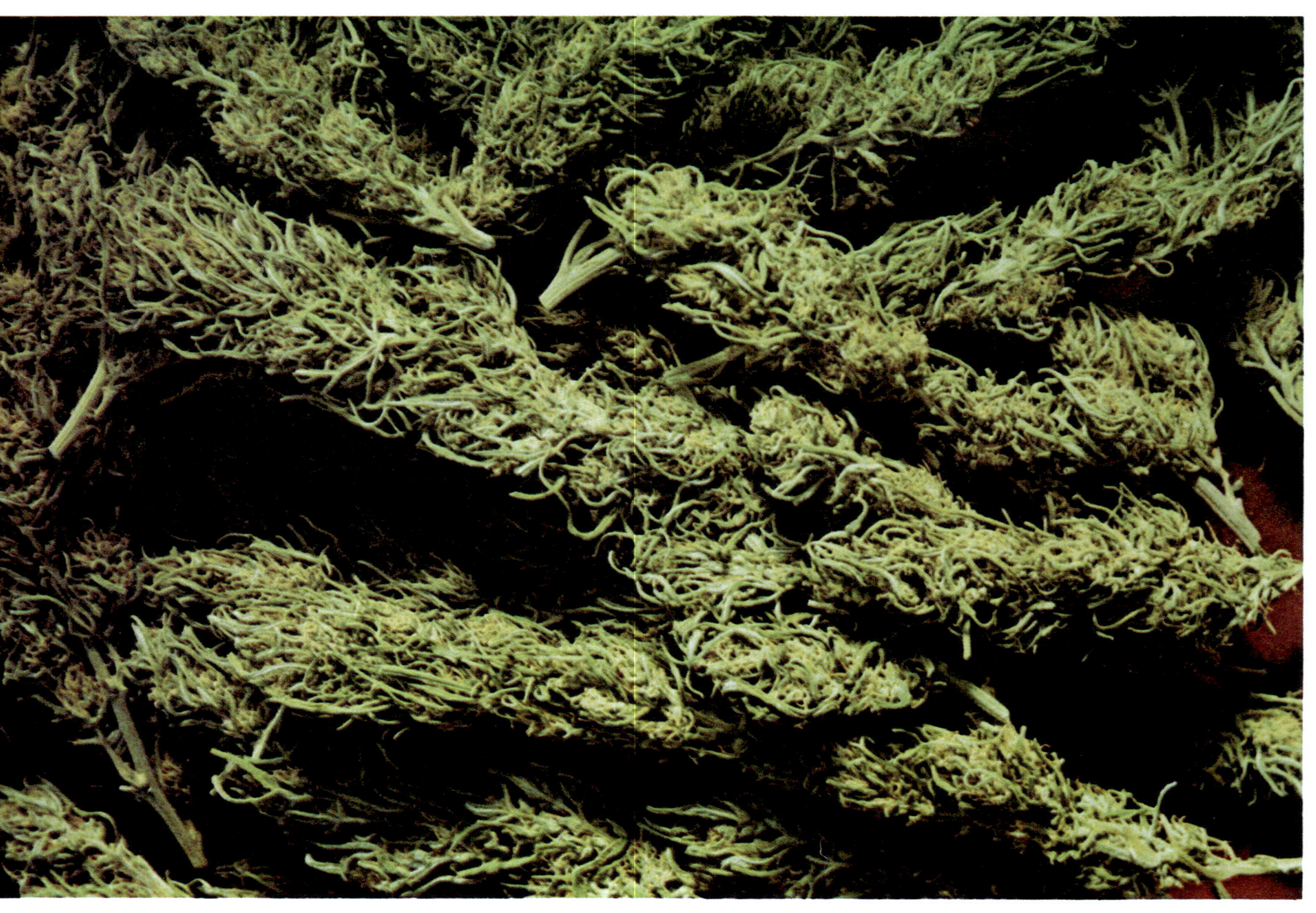

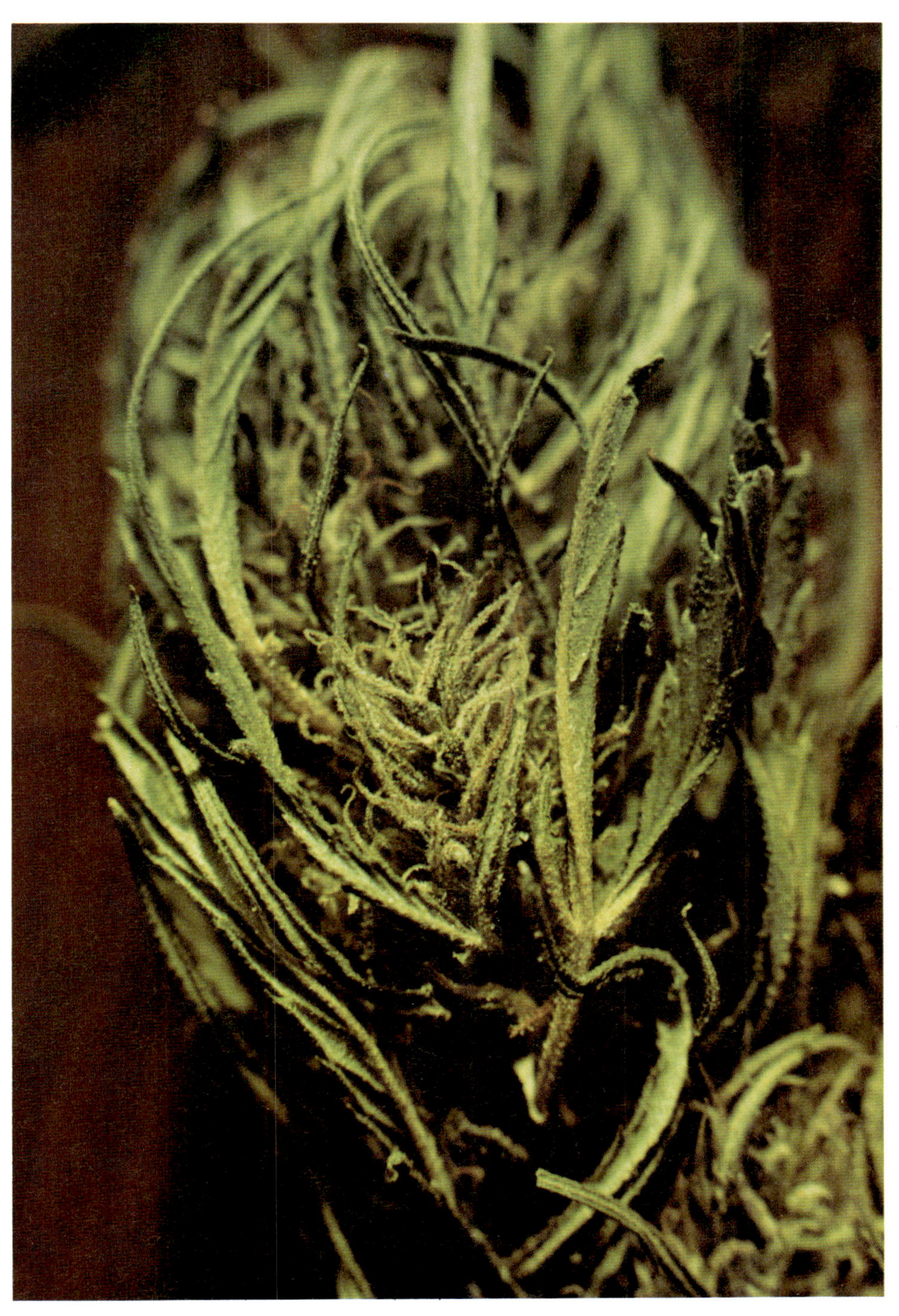

close-up of the dried colas

IN THE CURING PROCESS a sufficient amount of the natural moisture is removed from the flower clusters to prevent organic deterioration. There are many good methods of curing, but slow and gentle drying is best for any herb. Excessive heat may cook the flavor and potency out of the delicate flowers. Moisture allowed to absorb back into the fibres from the air can cause discoloration and mold. (For this reason, commercial marijuana is usually brown and musty.) When allowed to overdry, the flowers crumble into powder at the slightest touch. A point just short of this is best when the clusters are cured but not brittle. Storage should be air tight.

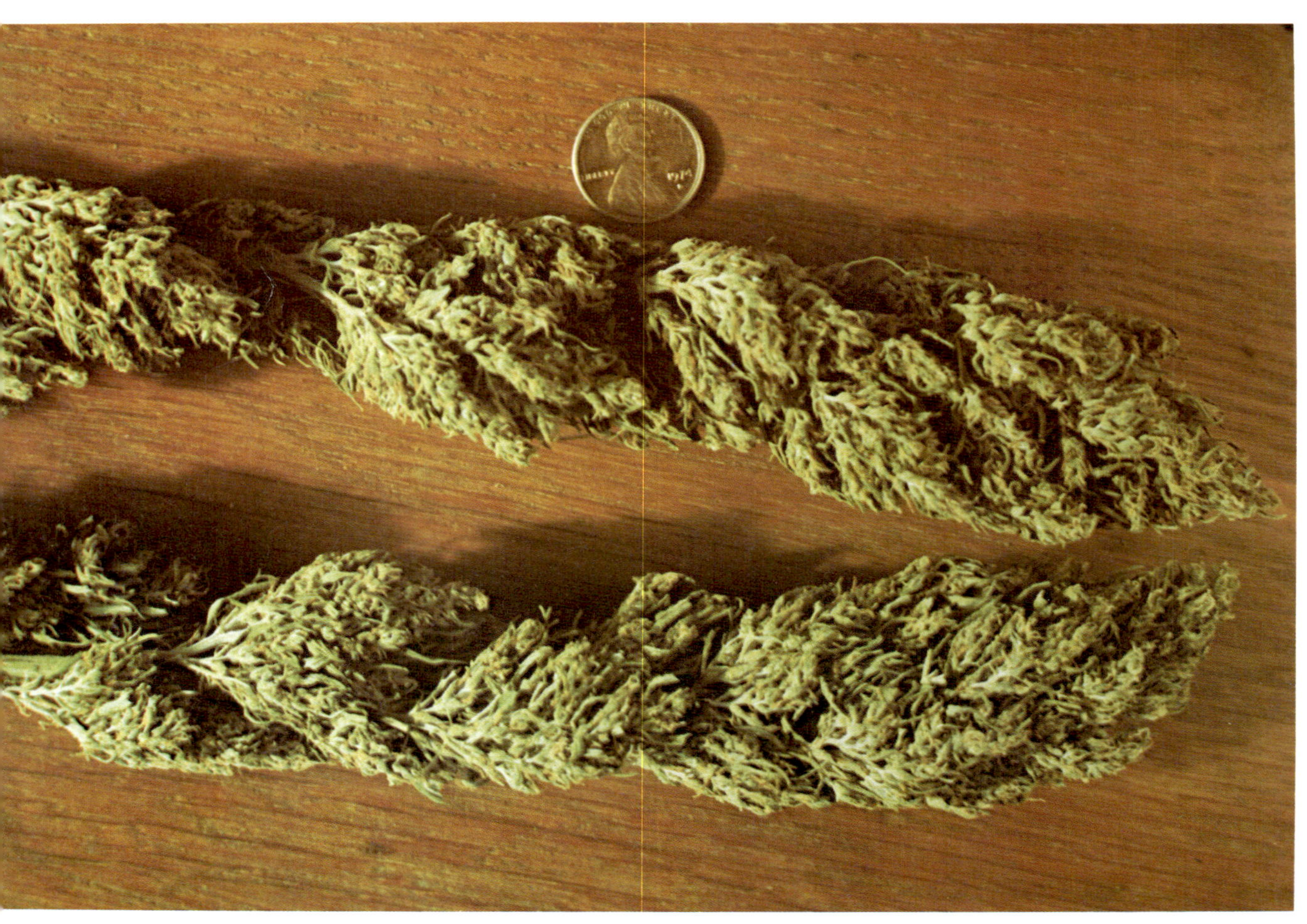

some large colas picked clean of superfluous
leaf—see live plant (pages 48, 49)

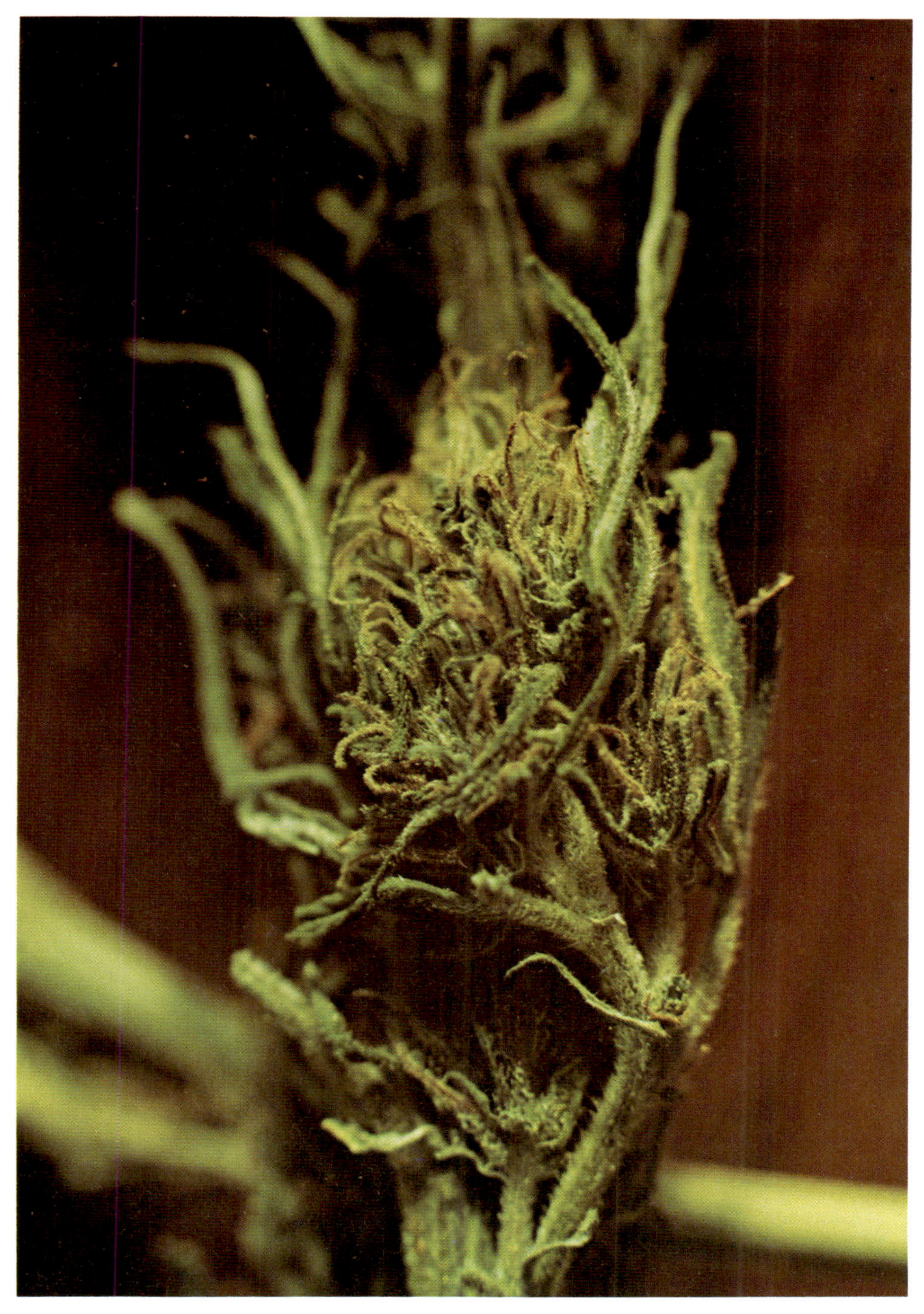

tight little clusters of blonde flowers

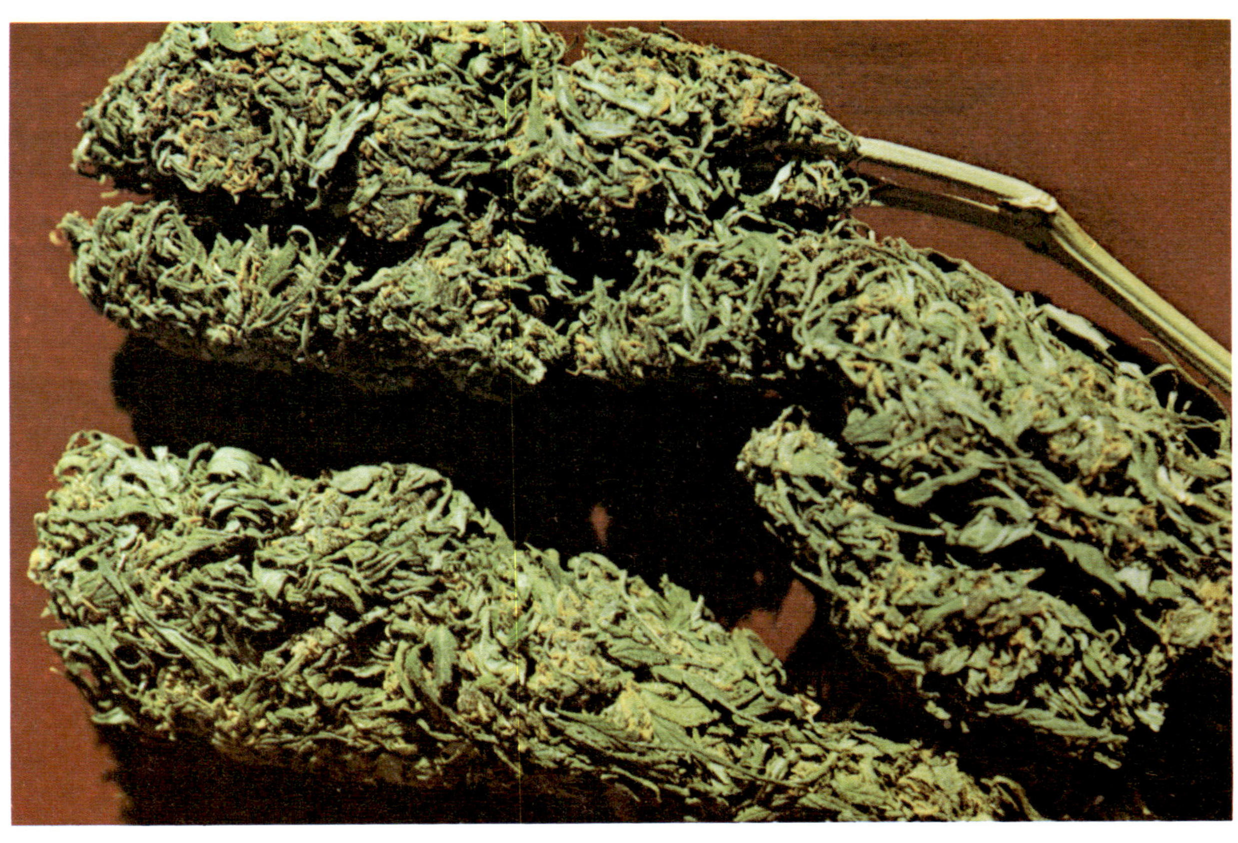

*some huge colas from a truly purple strain—the pistils dried a bright orange
these colas had occasional seeds*

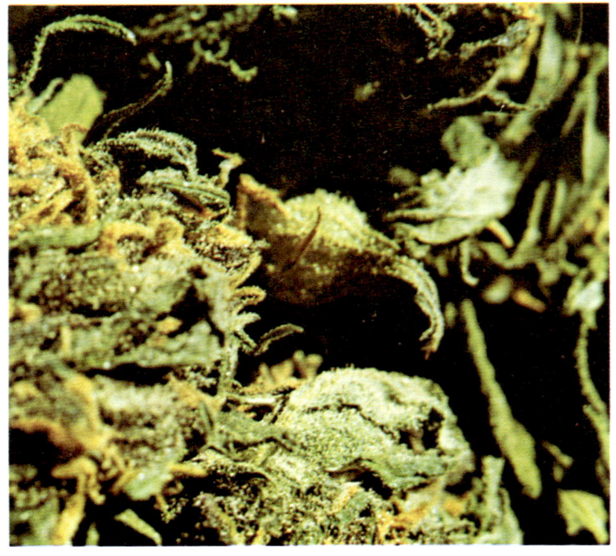

a single seed in the cluster

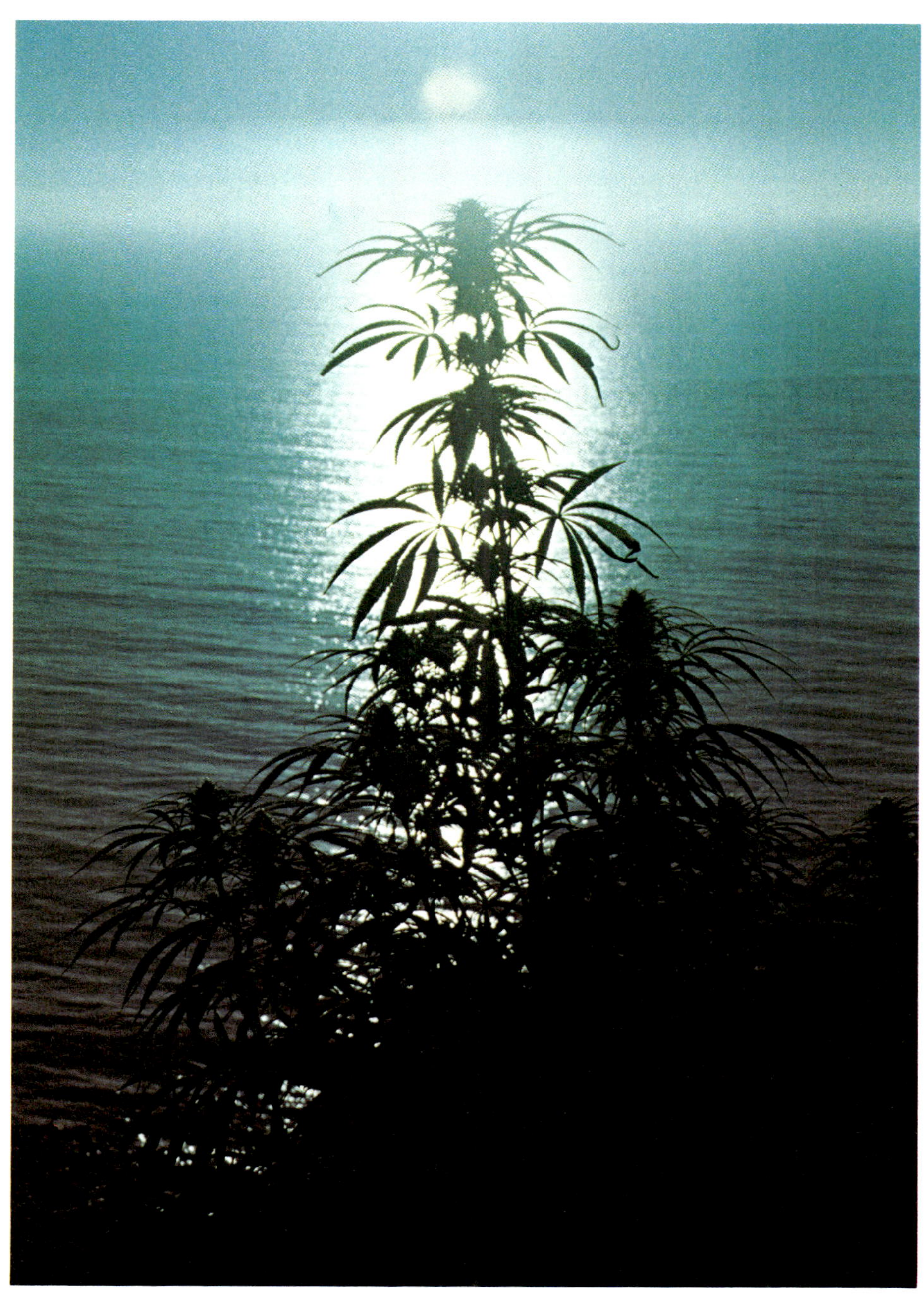

IN CONCLUSION we would like
to thank all those people who have
affirmed our experience with their
own, and who have helped refine
our presentation by openly admit-
ting us to their gardens and their
thoughts.

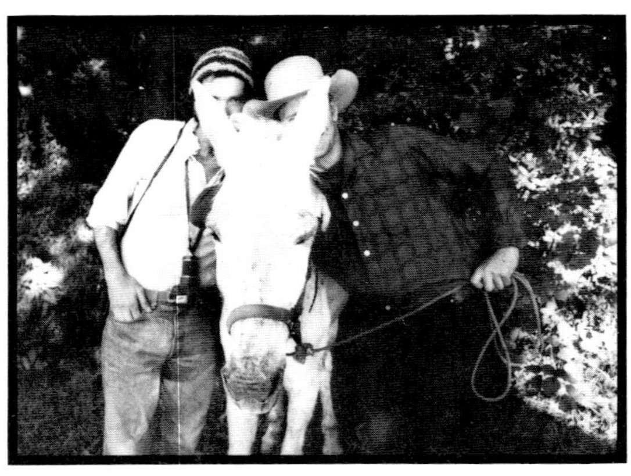

Incidental Notes

Text set in Tiffany; display faces are Vivaldi and York

*All exposures were made on Eastman 5254 Color Negative,
under available light conditions with 35mm Pentax equipment*

Illustration on page 4 by C. J. Panziera
Production layout by Kira Godbe
Design by Richardson & Woods